Oral Care in Advanced Disease

Oral Care in Advanced Disease

Edited by

Dr Andrew Davies
Consultant in Palliative Medicine
Royal Marsden Hospital, Sutton, UK

and

Professor Ilora Finlay
(Baroness Finlay of Llandaff)
Professor of Palliative Medicine
Cardiff University, Cardiff, UK

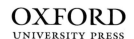

OXFORD
UNIVERSITY PRESS

This book has been printed digitally and produced in a standard specification
in order to ensure its continuing availability

OXFORD
UNIVERSITY PRESS

Great Clarendon Street, Oxford OX2 6DP

Oxford University Press is a department of the University of Oxford.
It furthers the University's objective of excellence in research, scholarship,
and education by publishing worldwide in

Oxford New York

Auckland Cape Town Dar es Salaam Hong Kong Karachi
Kuala Lumpur Madrid Melbourne Mexico City Nairobi
New Delhi Shanghai Taipei Toronto
With offices in
Argentina Austria Brazil Chile Czech Republic France Greece
Guatemala Hungary Italy Japan South Korea Poland Portugal
Singapore Switzerland Thailand Turkey Ukraine Vietnam

Oxford is a registered trade mark of Oxford University Press
in the UK and in certain other countries

Published in the United States
by Oxford University Press Inc., New York

ISBN 978-0-19-263243-2

Printed and bound by CPI Antony Rowe, Eastbourne

We would like to dedicate this book to our parents Diana and John Davies (A.D.), and Thaïs and Charles Downman (I.F.).

Preface

Oral problems are a major cause of morbidity in patients with advanced disease. Nevertheless, oral problems have assumed a low priority within palliative care, and other medical specialties. Moreover, the management of oral problems has often been based on historical anecdote, rather than on contemporary research.

We set out to produce an up-to-date, evidence-based, clinically relevant, user-friendly textbook on oral problems in patients with advanced disease. Unfortunately, in many instances, the evidence was not as robust as we would have wished. We hope that the book will encourage more healthcare professionals to undertake research into oral problems.

More importantly, we hope that the book will encourage all healthcare professionals to take the issue of oral hygiene and oral problems more seriously. Oral care should be the concern of the whole multidisciplinary team, rather than of the most junior nurses on the team. Indeed, it should be regarded as an essential aspect of the care of all patients with advanced disease.

We are indebted to our contributors, many of who contributed not only to their own chapter, but also to relevant sections of other authors' chapters. In particular, we are grateful to Professor Jeremy Bagg, Dr John Eveson and Dr Petrina Sweeney for providing many of the clinical photographs, and to Dr Anita Sengupta for commissioning all of the original artwork.

Finally, we would like to acknowledge the continual advice and support provided by Professor Jeremy Bagg, Dr Petrina Sweeney, and the staff at Oxford University Press.

A.D.
I.F.

Contents

Contributors

Jeremy Bagg
Professor of Clinical Microbiology
University of Glasgow Dental School
Glasgow, UK

David Beighton
Professor of Oral Microbiology
The Dental Institute
Kings College London
London, UK

Susan Brailsford
Honorary Postdoctoral Research Fellow
The Dental Institute
Kings College London
London, UK

Mark Chambers
Department of Head and Neck
Surgery/Radiation Oncology
MD Anderson Cancer Center
Houston, TX
USA

Andrew Davies
Consultant in Palliative Medicine
Royal Marsden Hospital
Sutton, UK

Louis DePaola
Department of Oral Medicine
and Diagnostic Sciences
Dental School
University of Maryland
Baltimore, MD
USA

John Eveson
Reader and Honorary Consultant in Oral
Medicine and Pathology
University of Bristol
Bristol, UK

Ilora Finlay
(Baroness Finlay of Llandaff)
Professor of Palliative Medicine
Cardiff University
Cardiff, UK

Janice Fiske
Senior Lecturer and Consultant in
Special Care Dentistry
The Dental Institute
Kings College London
London, UK

Fabio Fulfaro
Operative Unit of Medical Oncology
University of Palermo
Palermo
Italy

Adam Garden
Department of Radiation Oncology
MD Anderson Cancer Center
Houston, TX
USA

Richard Hain
Senior Lecturer in Paediatric Palliative
Medicine
Cardiff University
Cardiff, UK

Merrill Kies
Department of Thoracic/Head and Neck
Medical Oncology
MD Anderson Cancer Center
Houston, TX
USA

James Lemon
Department of Head and Neck Surgery
MD Anderson Cancer Center
Houston, TX
USA

Victoria Lucas
Senior Clinical Research Fellow
The Eastman Dental Institute
London, UK

Jack Martin
Department of Head and Neck Surgery
MD Anderson Cancer Center
Houston, TX
USA

John Meechan
Senior Lecturer and Honorary
Consultant in Oral and
Maxillofacial Surgery
The School of Dental Sciences
University of Newcastle
Newcastle upon Tyne, UK

Carla Ripamonti
Rehabilitation and Palliative Care
Operative Unit
National Cancer Institute of Milan
Milan
Italy

Graham Roberts
Professor of Paediatric Dentistry
The Eastman Dental Institute
London, UK

Jan Roodenburg
Department of Oral and Maxillofacial
Surgery
University Hospital
Groningen
The Netherlands

Anita Sengupta
Lecturer in Anatomy
University of Bristol
Bristol, UK

Kate Shorthose
Clinical Fellow in Oncology
Bristol Haematology and Oncology
Centre
Bristol, UK

Arley Silva
Assistant Professor of Stomatology
Dental School
Gama Filho University
Rio de Janeiro
Brazil

Petrina Sweeney
Clinical Senior Lecturer in Adult Special
Needs Dentistry
University of Glasgow Dental School
Glasgow, UK

Angus Walls
Professor of Restorative Dentistry
The School of Dental Sciences
University of Newcastle
Newcastle upon Tyne, UK

Chapter 1

Introduction

Andrew Davies

Introduction

The aim of this chapter is to provide an introduction to oral problems in patients with advanced disease. The majority of people receiving specialist palliative care are patients with advanced cancer. Thus the emphasis of the chapter will be on studies involving this group of patients.

Epidemiology

Oral symptoms are common in palliative care patients (Table 1.1).[1–4] Most patients have at least one symptom, and many patients have several.[2,4] Oral symptoms are also common relative to other symptoms in palliative care patients (Table 1.2).[4] Indeed, dry mouth (xerostomia) is consistently ranked as one of the five most common symptoms in patients with advanced cancer.[5–8]

Oral infections are also common in palliative care patients. There have been a number of studies that have looked at oral candidosis in this group (Table 1.3).[1,2,9–12] In contrast, few studies have looked at other oral infections in this group. Nevertheless, active dental caries has been reported in 20–35 per cent of patients[2,3], and active gingivitis in 36 per cent patients.[1] Other oral infections are probably less common.

Aetiology

Oral problems may be related to:

- Direct effect of the primary disease
- Indirect effect of the primary disease (see below)
- Treatment of the primary disease
- Direct/indirect effect of a coexisting disease
- Treatment of the coexisting disease
- Combination of the above factors.

One of the most important causes of oral problems is the indirect effect of the primary disease. Thus, as the disease progresses, the patient becomes increasingly disabled, and increasingly less able to maintain oral hygiene. Other relevant factors

Table 1.1 Prevalence of oral symptoms in palliative care patients

Study	Population type/size	Prevalence oral symptoms					
		Dry mouth (%)	Oral discomfort (%)	Taste disturbance (%)	Difficulty chewing (%)	Difficulty swallowing (%)	Difficulty speaking (%)
Gordon et al. 1985 [1]	Hospice inpatients (N=31)	62	55	31	52	No data	59
Aldred et al. 1991 [2]	Hospice inpatients (N=20)	58	42	26	No data	37	No data
Jobbins et al. 1992 [3]	Hospice inpatients (N=197)	77	33	37	No data	35	No data
Davies 2000 [4]	Hospital support team patients (N=120)	78	46	44	23	23	31

Table 1.2 Prevalence of all symptoms in a palliative care population[4]

Symptom	Palliative care population $N = 120$ (%)
Lack of energy	109 (91)
Feeling drowsy	101 (84)
Pain	95 (79)
Dry mouth	93 (78)
Worrying	74 (62)
Constipation	71 (59)
Nausea	70 (58)
Shortness of breath	69 (58)
Lack of appetite	68 (57)
Difficulty concentrating	66 (55)
Feeling bloated	64 (53)
Difficulty sleeping	63 (53)
Feeling sad	61 (51)
Mouth discomfort	55 (46)
Change in the way food tastes	53 (44)
Feeling nervous	52 (43)
Feeling irritable	52 (43)
Sweats	51 (43)
Vomiting	48 (40)
Swelling of arms or legs	47 (39)
Numbness/tingling in hands/feet	46 (38)
Cough	44 (37)
Dizziness	43 (36)
Weight loss	38 (32)
Difficulty speaking	37 (31)
Problems with urination	35 (29)
'I don't look like myself'	34 (28)
Itching	32 (27)
Diarrhoea	31 (26)
Changes in skin	31 (26)
Difficulty swallowing	28 (23)
Difficulty chewing	27 (23)
Problems with sexual interest or activity	21 (18)
Mouth sores	17 (14)
Hair loss	14 (12)

Table 1.3 Prevalence of oral candidosis in patients with advanced cancer

Study	Population type/size	Prevalence of oral candidosis (%)
Boggs et al. 1961[9]	Hospital inpatient (N=90)	14
Rodu et al. 1984[10]	Hospital inpatient (N=52)	8
Gordon et al. 1985[1]	Hospice inpatient (N=31)	10
Clarke et al. 1987[11]	Hospice inpatient (N=46)	83
Aldred et al. 1991[2]	Hospice inpatient (N = 20)	70
Davies et al. 2001[12]	Hospital support team patients (N=120)	30

may be accompanying psychological disturbance and accompanying cognitive impairment. Another very important cause of oral problems is the treatment of the primary disease. Indeed, many of the treatments used to manage cancer, and many of the treatments used to manage the symptoms of cancer, can cause oral problems.

Clinical features

It is not unusual for patients to experience multiple oral problems during their illness. Furthermore, it is not unusual for patients to experience multiple oral problems at any one time during their illness. Such problems are common during the active treatment phase of the illness, and particularly during the terminal phase of the illness. They may be transient, intermittent, or persistent.

Oral problems are a significant cause of morbidity in palliative care patients. Table 1.4 shows the severity of oral symptoms, whilst Table 1.5 shows the distress caused by oral symptoms, in a palliative care population.[4] Oral problems can lead to a more generalized deterioration in a patient's physical state, and also in their psychological state.[13]

Table 1.4 Severity of oral symptoms in a palliative care population[4]

Symptom (N=120)	Slight (%)	Moderate (%)	Severe (%)	Very severe (%)
Dry mouth (N=93)	14	37	33	16
Mouth discomfort (N=55)	40	29	22	9
Change in the way food tastes (N=53)	30	45	19	6
Difficulty speaking (N=37)	40	30	19	11
Difficulty swallowing (N=28)	46	29	14	11
Difficulty chewing (N=27)	41	41	11	7
Mouth sores (N=17)	59	35	6	0

Table 1.5 Distress caused by oral symptoms in a palliative care population[4]

Symptom (*N* = 120)	Not at all (%)	A little bit (%)	Somewhat (%)	Quite a bit (%)	Very much (%)
Dry mouth (*N* = 93)	16	21	23	26	14
Mouth discomfort (*N* = 55)	16	31	18	26	9
Change in the way food tastes (*N* = 53)	17	32	23	21	7
Difficulty speaking (*N* = 37)	3	32	24	22	19
Difficulty swallowing (*N* = 28)	11	28	36	14	11
Difficulty chewing (*N* = 27)	11	44	15	30	0
Mouth sores (*N* = 17)	18	35	18	29	0

Management

The management of any oral problem involves:

- Adequate assessment of the oral problem
- Treatment of the underlying cause of the oral problem
- Active treatment of the oral problem ('cure')
- Symptomatic treatment of the oral problem ('palliation').

As mentioned above, many patients suffer from persistent oral problems: these are usually the result of inadequate treatment of the condition. Similarly, many patients suffer from recurrent oral problems: these are usually the result of inadequate treatment of the underlying cause. It should be noted that some 'standard' palliative care interventions for oral problems are ineffective/inappropriate for those oral problems.[14–16]

Multidisciplinary working

Dental professionals are important members of the extended palliative care team.[17] They have a number of key roles, including (a) training of palliative care professionals; (b) management of complex oral problems; and (c) management of specific oral problems.

Many dental procedures can be performed in the domiciliary setting, such as dental restorations and denture alterations (see Chapter 4).[18] However, domiciliary dentistry requires specialized skills, and appropriate resources/equipment.

It should be noted that other members of the multidisciplinary team might also have a role in the management of certain oral problems (for example speech and language therapists and dieticians).

References

1. Gordon SR, Berkey DB, Call RL (1985). Dental need among hospice patients in Colorado: a pilot study. *Gerodontics* **1**: 125–9.

2. Aldred MJ, Addy M, Bagg J, Finlay I (1991). Oral health in the terminally ill: a cross-sectional pilot survey. *Spec Care Dentist* **11**: 59–62.

3. Jobbins J, Bagg J, Finlay IG, Addy M, Newcombe RG (1992). Oral and dental disease in terminally ill cancer patients. *BMJ* **304**: 1612.

4. Davies ANT (2000). An investigation into the relationship between salivary gland hypofunction and oral health problems in patients with advanced cancer. Dissertation King's College: University of London.

5. Reuben DB, Mor V, Hiris J (1988). Clinical symptoms and length of survival in patients with terminal cancer. *Arch Intern Med* **148**: 1586–91.

6. Dunlop GM (1989). A study of the relative frequency and importance of gastrointestinal symptoms, and weakness in patients with far advanced cancer: student paper. *Palliat Med* **4**: 37–43.

7. Ventafridda V, De Conno F, Ripamonti C, Gamba A, Tamburini M (1990). Quality-of-life assessment during a palliative care programme. *Ann Oncol* **1**: 415–20.

8. Curtis EB, Krech R, Walsh TD (1991). Common symptoms in patients with advanced cancer. *J Palliat Care* **7**: 25–9.

9. Boggs DR, Williams AF, Howell A (1961). Thrush in malignant neoplastic disease. *Arch Intern Med* **107**: 354–60.

10. Rodu B, Griffin IL, Gockerman JP (1984). Oral candidosis in cancer patients. *Southern Med J* **77**: 312–14.

11. Clarke JMG, Wilson JA, von Haacke NP, Milne LJR (1987). Oral candidiasis in terminal illness. *Health Bull (Edinb)* **45**: 268–71.

12. Davies AN, Brailsford S, Beighton D (2001). Corticosteroids and oral candidosis. *Palliat Med* **15**: 521.

13. Rydholm M, Strang P (2002). Physical and psychosocial impact of xerostomia in palliative cancer care: a qualitative interview study. *Int J Palliat Nurs* **8**: 318–23.

14. Regnard C, Allport S, Stephenson L (1997). ABC of palliative care. Mouth care, skin care, and lymphoedema. *BMJ* **315**: 1002–05.

15. Davies A (1998). Clinically proven treatments for xerostomia were ignored. *BMJ* **316**: 1247.

16. Pemberton M, Thornhill MH (1998). Simple antiseptic mouthwashes are best for infection. *BMJ* **316**: 1247.

17. Cummings I (1998). The interdisciplinary team. In D Doyle, GWC Hanks, N MacDonald (ed.) *Oxford Textbook of Palliative Medicine*, 2nd edn. p. 21. Oxford: Oxford University Press.

18. Walls AWG, Murray ID (1993). Dental care of patients in hospice. *Palliat Med* **7**: 313–21.

Chapter 2

Oral assessment

Andrew Davies

Introduction

The assessment of oral problems is essentially similar to the assessment of other medical problems. It involves taking a history, performing an examination, and the use of appropriate investigations.[1]

History

The standard medical history involves a superficial assessment of oral symptoms. However, as discussed in Chapter 1, oral problems are particularly common in palliative care patients. Therefore, a more thorough oral history should be taken in this group of patients.

The oral history should include questions about the following symptoms:

- Oral discomfort/pain
- Dry mouth (xerostomia)
- Taste disturbance
- Difficulty chewing (dysmasesia)
- Difficulty swallowing (dysphagia)
- Difficulty speaking (dysphonia)
- Bad breath (halitosis)
- Drooling.

This list includes the most common oral symptoms experienced by palliative care patients.[2,3] However, patients may experience other oral symptoms. Thus, patients should be encouraged to report 'any other problems' relating to the oral cavity. Patients with dental prostheses should be asked specifically about associated problems (discomfort, poor fitting).

It is often insufficient to simply ask about the presence of a symptom. The format of additional questioning will depend on the nature of the symptom. For example, questions about pain should include:

- onset
- temporal pattern

- site
- radiation
- quality/character
- intensity/severity
- exacerbating factors
- relieving factors
- response to analgesics
- associated symptoms, and
- interference with activities of daily living.[4]

The extent of additional questioning will depend on a variety of factors, including the nature of the symptom and the general health of the patient.

It is important to ask about the presence of oral symptoms, because patients do not always volunteer information about them. The reasons for this phenomenon are undetermined. However, one factor is likely to be the relative lack of importance healthcare professionals attach to oral problems.[5] Thus, Kutner *et al.* reported that hospice staff often could not comment on the presence or absence of oral symptoms in their patients.[6]

Examination

The standard medical examination involves an assessment of oral signs, although this is usually with the aim of identifying systemic diseases, rather of than identifying oral diseases. For the reasons stated above, a more thorough oral examination should be performed in this group of patients.

The oral examination involves general observation, intra-oral examination, and extra-oral examination (lymph nodes, salivary glands).[1] The techniques used to examine the interior of the oral cavity include: (a) inspection; (b) palpation; and (c) olfaction. The main technique is inspection. Inspection is primarily used to assess structure, although it is also used to assess function (movement).

The examination should be conducted with the patient either seated in a chair, or lying on a bed. It is advantageous to have good background light source, but essential to have a good direct light source (torch). A spatula, or gloved finger, should be used to aid inspection of the oral cavity. Moreover, a gloved finger should be used to palpate relevant oral lesions.

The examination should begin with any dental prostheses *in situ*, but should continue with the dental prostheses removed. It is important to examine the patient with their dental prostheses *in situ* in order to assess fitting. However, it is equally important to examine the patient with their dental prostheses removed, since it may be concealing oral pathology (Figs 2.1(a) and (b)).

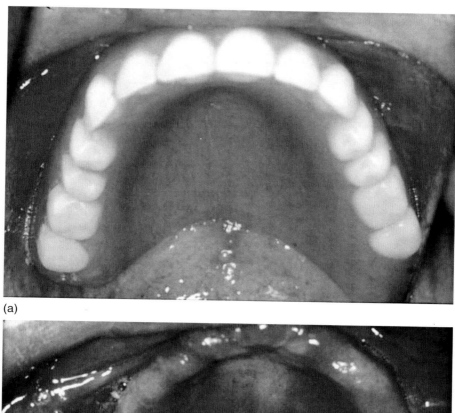

(a)

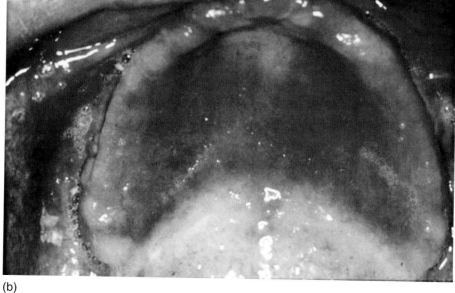

(b)

Fig. 2.1 (a) Denture *in situ* (no obvious oral pathology). **(b)** Denture removed, revealing denture stomatitis. Both are reproduced with permission from M. P. Sweeney and J. Bagg (1997), *Making Sense of the Mouth*, Partnership in Oral Care, Glasgow. (See also Plates 1(a) and (b) at the centre of this book.)

The oral cavity needs to be examined systematically (Fig. 2.2).[1]:

- Upper/lower labial sulci – retract the upper/lower lip.
- Buccal mucosa and upper/lower buccal sulci on right side – retract the right cheek.
- Buccal mucosa and upper/lower buccal sulci on left side – retract the left cheek.
- Dorsal surface of tongue – ask the patient to stick out their tongue.
- Ventral surface of tongue – ask the patient to raise their tongue upwards. The motor function of the tongue can be assessed by asking the patient to move their tongue from side to side.
- Floor of mouth – ask the patient to raise their tongue upwards.
- Hard/soft palate – the motor function of the soft palate can be assessed by asking the patient to say 'Ah'.
- Teeth.

The format/extent of the examination will depend on a variety factors, including the diagnosis of the patient, and the general health of the patient. For example, patients with chronic neurological diseases, and some patients with advanced cancer, require a more thorough neurological examination.[7]

Figures 2.3–2.6 demonstrate the normal (healthy) appearance of the mouth. Similarly, Figs 2.7 and 2.8 demonstrate the normal (usual) anatomy of the mouth. The terminology of oral mucosal lesions is shown in Table 2.1.

Investigations

A wide range of investigations is used in Oral Medicine.[1] Some of these investigations are of relevance to Palliative Care, e.g. microbiological testing. The decision to perform an investigation will depend on the nature of the problem (unimportant, important), the nature of the investigation (invasive, non-invasive), the likely outcome of the investigation (management unaltered, management altered), and the general health of the patient. The role of specific investigations is discussed in subsequent chapters.

Assessment tools

Oral assessment tools are widely used in Palliative Care. A variety of oral assessment tools have been developed. This section discusses oral assessment tools, which are of specific relevance to Palliative Care, i.e. the Oral Assessment Guide[8] and the Heals' tool.[9]

The Oral Assessment Guide was developed for use in patients with mucositis secondary to chemotherapy and/or radiotherapy (Table 2.2).[8] It was found to be reliable (inter-observer reliability), and felt to have validity (content validity) in this setting. The tool was used to determine the frequency of oral intervention, i.e. the worse the oral score, the more frequent the oral intervention.

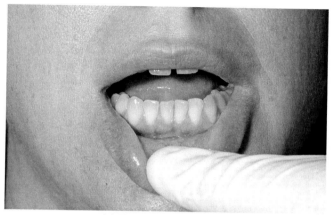

(a) Retract the lower lip.

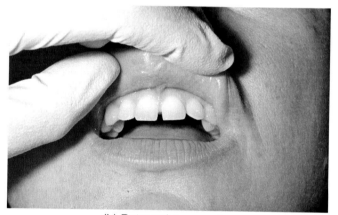

(b) Retract the upper lip.

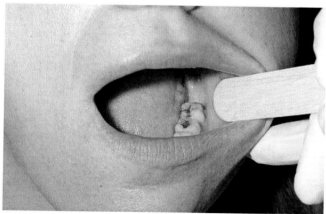

(c) Retract the left cheek (upper/lower part).

Fig. 2.2 Technique of oral examination.

(*Continued*)

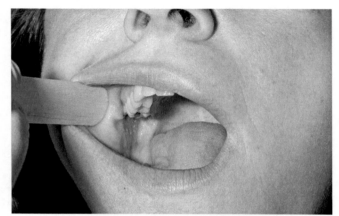

(d) Retract the right cheek (upper/lower part).

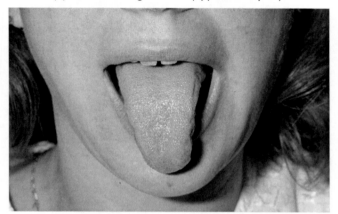

(e) Ask patient to stick out their tongue.

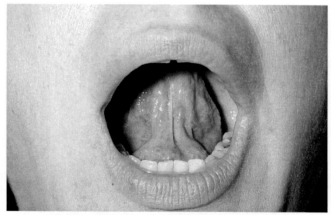

(f) Ask patient to raise their tongue upwards.

Fig. 2.2 Cont'd

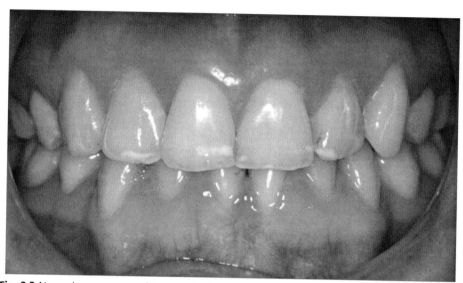

Fig. 2.3 Normal appearance of the gingiva/teeth. Courtesy of J. Eveson. (See also Plate 2 at the centre of this book.)

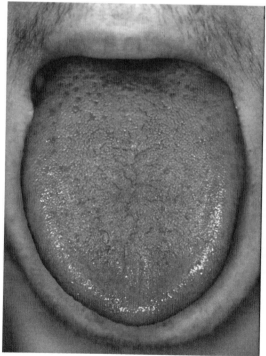

Fig. 2.4 Normal appearance of the tongue. Courtesy of J. Eveson. (See also Plate 3 at the centre of this book.)

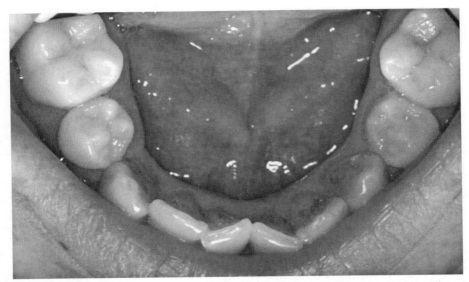

Fig. 2.5 Normal appearance of the floor of the mouth. Courtesy of J. Eveson. (See also Plate 4 at the centre of this book.)

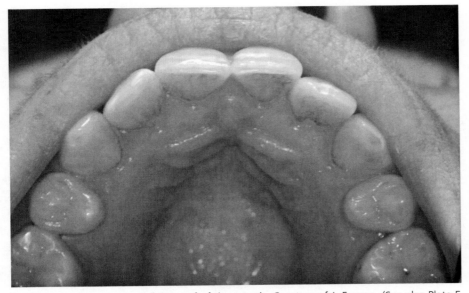

Fig. 2.6 Normal appearance of the roof of the mouth. Courtesy of J. Eveson. (See also Plate 5 at the centre of this book.)

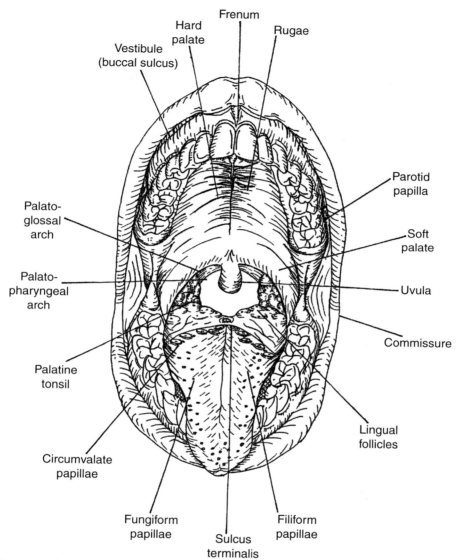

Fig. 2.7 Anatomy of the mouth. Courtesy of the Department of Anatomy, University of Bristol.

The Oral Assessment Guide has been investigated in patients with advanced cancer.[10] It was not found to be completely reliable, and was not felt to have complete validity in this setting. However, it was felt to be superior to other tested oral assessment tools. In spite of its limitations, the Oral Assessment Guide has been recommended for use in patients with advanced cancer.[11]

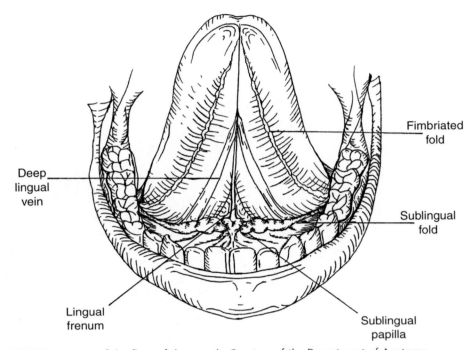

Fig. 2.8 Anatomy of the floor of the mouth. Courtesy of the Department of Anatomy, University of Bristol.

Table 2.1 Terminology of oral mucosal lesions[1]

Term	Description
Erythema	Red colouration
Erosion	Partial thickness loss of epithelium (underlying connective tissue not exposed)
Ulcer	Full thickness loss of epithelium (underlying connective tissue exposed)
Papule	Small, well-defined, elevated area
Plaque	Large, well-defined, elevated area
Vesicle	Well-defined accumulation of fluid within/beneath epithelium (< 5mm in diameter)
Bulla	Well-defined accumulation of fluid within/beneath epithelium (> 5mm in diameter)
Sinus	Blind-ending tract
Fistula	Connecting tract (between two epithelial surfaces)

Table 2.2 The Oral Assessment Guide. Adapted from reference [8]

	Numerical and descriptive ratings		
Category	**1**	**2**	**3**
Voice	Normal	Deeper or raspy	Difficulty talking or painful
Swallow	Normal swallow	Some pain on swallow	Unable to swallow
Lips	Smooth and pink and moist	Dry or cracked	Ulcerated or bleeding
Tongue	Pink and moist and papillae present	Coated or loss of papillae with a shiny appearance with or without redness	Blistered or cracked
Saliva	Watery	Thick or ropy	Absent
Mucous membranes	Pink and moist	Reddened or coated (increased whiteness) without ulcerations	Ulcerations with or without bleeding
Gingiva	Pink and stippled and firm	Oedematous with or without redness	Spontaneous bleeding or bleeding with pressure
Teeth or dentures (or denture bearing area)	Clean and no debris	Plaque or debris in localized areas (between teeth if present)	Plaque or debris generalized along gum line or denture-bearing area

The Heals' tool was specifically developed for use in patients with advanced cancer.[9] It does not appear to have been formally evaluated. Despite this omission, the Heals' tool has been used as a research outcome measure.[12] It should be noted that the researchers made adaptations to the tool, because of concerns about its validity.[12]

As discussed above, the major problem with oral assessment tools is their lack of validity. Thus, the tools often fail to assess common oral problems. For example, the Oral Assessment Guide[8] does not assess oral discomfort/pain, taste distur-bance, difficulty chewing, bad breath, or drooling. Similarly, the tools often fail to adequately assess common oral problems. For example, the Oral Assessment Guide[8] does not assess subjective symptoms of salivary gland dysfunction. (Patients with salivary gland dysfunction may have subjective symptoms, but may not have objective signs.)

Another major problem with oral assessment tools is their end point. Oral assessment tools produce a score, rather than a diagnosis. A poor score implies that some type of intervention is required, but does not determine what that inter-vention should be. A poor score is usually associated with significant oral pathology. Conversely, significant oral pathology is not always associated with a poor score. For example, a patient with oral candidosis may only score 9/24 on the Oral Assessment Guide (2/3 in the mucous membrane category; 1/3 in the other categories).[8]

On the basis of the above, there seems little justification for the routine use of oral assessment tools in the palliative care setting.

References

1. Birnbaum W, Dunne SM (2000). *Oral Diagnosis: the clinician's guide*. Oxford: Wright.
2. Gordon SR, Berkey DB, Call RL (1985). Dental need among hospice patients in Colorado: a pilot study. *Gerodontics* 1: 125–9.
3. Aldred MJ, Addy M, Bagg J, Finlay I (1991). Oral health in the terminally ill: a cross-sectional pilot survey. *Spec Care Dentist* 11: 59–62.
4. Foley KM (1998). Pain assessment and cancer pain syndromes. In D Doyle, GW Hanks, N MacDonald (ed.) *Oxford Textbook of Palliative Medicine*, 2nd edn, pp. 310–31. Oxford: Oxford University Press.
5. Senn HJ (1997). Orphan topics in supportive care: how about xerostomia? *Support Care Cancer* 5: 261–2.
6. Kutner JS, Kassner CT, Nowels DE (2001). Symptom burden at the end of life: hospice providers' experience. *J Pain Symptom Manage* 21: 473–80.
7. Cull RE, Whittle IR (2000). The nervous system. In JF Munro, IW Campbell (ed.) *Macleod's Clinical Examination*, 10th edn, pp. 196–214. Edinburgh: Churchill Livingstone.
8. Eilers J, Berger A, Petersen M (1988). Development, testing and application of the oral assessment guide. *Oncol Nurs Forum* 15: 325–30.
9. Heals D (1993). A key to well-being: oral hygiene in patients with advanced cancer. *Prof Nurse* 8: 391–8.

10. Holmes S, Mountain E (1993). Assessment of oral status: evaluation of three oral assessment guides. *J Clin Nurs* **2**: 35–40.

11. Anonymous (1996). *Managing Oral Care Problems Throughout the Cancer Illness Trajectory*, pp. 7–11. London: The Macmillan Practice Development Unit.

12. Milligan S, McGill M, Sweeney MP, Malarkey C (2001). Oral care for patients with advanced cancer: an evidence-based protocol. *Int J Palliat Nurs* **7**: 418–26.

Chapter 3

Oral hygiene

Petrina Sweeney

Introduction

Maintenance of oral hygiene is important for all groups of patients, especially patients with advanced disease. Poor oral hygiene can have physical, psychological, and social consequences.[1] For example, poor oral hygiene may cause halitosis, which may result in the patient becoming depressed, and also in the family/friends becoming more distant. Poor oral hygiene can lead to other oral problems (e.g. dental caries), and also to certain systemic problems (e.g. aspiration pneumonia).[2] Clearly the maintenance of oral hygiene is important for the maintenance of quality of life.

Oral care – issues
Assessment of oral hygiene

A thorough oral assessment is the vital first step in planning effective care.[3,4] However, the assessment of oral health status is a largely neglected area of practice.[5] Without such an assessment, it is not possible to establish a baseline for, nor to evaluate the effectiveness of, oral care.[6] Oral assessment is discussed in detail in Chapter 2.

Maintenance of oral hygiene

Oral hygiene procedures need not be difficult, or time consuming. Patients should be encouraged to carry out, or participate in, their own oral care if at all possible. Some may require assistance with particular aspects of mouth care, or they may be completely dependent on others for all aspects of oral hygiene.

Specific, practical protocols can be developed dependent on the dental status of patients, but there are two central themes, namely regularity of assessment, and frequency of care. Examination of the mouth should take place daily to enable early detection and treatment of oral problems. Oral hygiene measures should be performed at least twice per day, if they are to benefit the patient. They must assume equal priority with other aspects of care, and be documented as part of individual care plans.

Active involvement of the dental profession is an essential part of the multidisciplinary approach required in effective palliative care.[7] Those nursing patients with advanced disease should attempt to organize appropriate input from a dental surgeon, who, in turn, can involve other members of the dental team, in particular a dental hygienist. The dental staff will carry out appropriate corrective measures, but it remains the responsibility of the nursing staff to provide regular oral care for patients.

Staff training

Oral health procedures are often given low priority compared to other care tasks performed by nursing and care staff.[8] Reasons for the low priority afforded to oral care include a lack of understanding and awareness of oral health problems, and the absence of standardized training in this area for all members of the medical team.[9–11] Oral care must be given higher priority in the education of nurses and care-workers, and should include basic information on dental disease and an explanation of the rationale behind oral hygiene procedures, if oral care is to reach an acceptable standard.[12]

Oral care – practice

General principles

Oral hygiene procedures should always be carried out in a gentle and dignified manner. Patients should be in a comfortable position, and should have their desire for privacy respected. For example, many people find it embarrassing to remove their dentures in public, and feel very uncomfortable when their dentures are outside the mouth.

Disposable medical gloves must always be worn when working in the mouth, or when handling items such as dentures. Similarly, the potential for transmission of micro-organisms between patients must be considered, and universal infection control procedures employed at all times.

Dental care

Toothbrushing

The single most important oral hygiene measure is toothbrushing, which should be undertaken at least twice daily.

Table 3.1 Oral care procedures for dentate patients

Procedure	Comments
Clean teeth at least twice daily	Use a personal toothbrush and a fluoridated toothpaste Carers must undertake tooth-brushing for dependent patients
Chemical plaque control	Consider using chlorhexidine mouthwash, spray, or gel
Maintain cleanliness of oral mucosa	Clean mucosa with a water-moistened gauze or a foam stick (if necessary)
Clean partial denture at least daily	See Table 3.2
Maintain complex dental work	The dental team should provide advice on oral hygiene for patients with complex restorations e.g. implants, crowns and bridges

Table 3.2 Oral care procedures for edentulous patients

Procedure	Comments
Clean denture at least daily	Use a personal brush and soap/water (clean dentures over water)
	Carers must undertake denture cleaning for dependent patients
	Dentures should be rinsed after meals
Remove/sterilize dentures at night	Plastic dentures may be soaked in either dilute sodium hypochlorite, or chlorhexidine
	Dentures with metal parts should be soaked in chlorhexidine
	Dentures should be rinsed after sterilization
Maintain cleanliness of oral mucosa	Clean mucosa with a water-moistened gauze or a foam stick (if necessary)
Mark denture with patient's name	See Table 3.3
	Kits are commercially available
Maintain dentures	Check dentures regularly for missing teeth, cracks and sharp edges

A wide range of toothbrushes is available commercially, including powered tooth-brushes (electric toothbrushes). It is recommended that a small-headed brush, which has medium texture, nylon filament bristles is used. Soft toothbrushes can be used for patients whose mouths are particularly sore. These toothbrushes include baby brushes and specialist brushes (e.g. the TePe® Special Care toothbrush). The recommended life of a toothbrush is approximately three months, but it should be replaced sooner if the filaments of the brush head become softened and misshapen. (At this stage the brush is no longer effective at removing plaque.) Toothbrushes should also be replaced if the patient has suffered a serious oral infection. Attention should be paid to the handle, which can be easily adapted to allow a firmer grip for those with problems of manual dexterity (Fig. 3.1). The local Occupational Therapy department should be able to offer advice on adaptive aids for toothbrushes, some of which are available commercially.

A recent systematic review has reported that the majority of powered toothbrushes are no better at removing plaque than manual toothbrushes.[13] However, patients who are accustomed to using a powered toothbrush should be encouraged to continue with it. Patients whose disability prevents them from using a manual toothbrush satisfactorily may also benefit from a powered toothbrush. Appropriate staff training is essential before using a powered toothbrush to provide oral care for another, as the oral and dental tissues are fragile and easily traumatized if excess force is used. Studies have shown that many nurses prefer to use a foam swab to clean a patient's teeth.[14,15] However, toothbrushes are recognized as being significantly more effective than foam swabs for removal of plaque from teeth.[16]

There are many brands of toothpaste available commercially. Patients should be encouraged to use toothpaste containing at least 1000 ppm fluoride. In addition to its anti-caries activity, fluoride also reduces dentine hypersensitivity, which can become an extremely troublesome symptom in patients with a dry mouth.[17] Most toothpastes

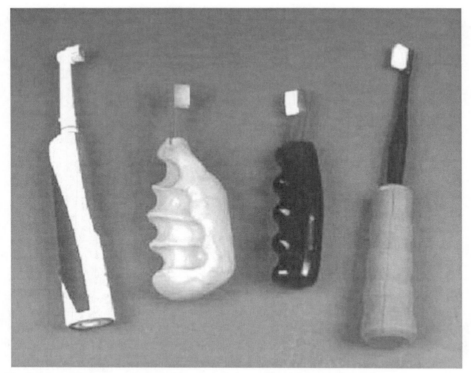

Fig. 3.1 An ordinary powered toothbrush and three adapted manual toothbrushes.

contain a foaming agent, which may prove problematic for those patients who have difficulty rinsing their mouths or swallowing, and who are at increased risk of aspiration. In these cases, a non-foaming alternative such as chlorhexidine gluconate gel should be used.[18] If patients cannot tolerate the use of toothpaste, because of discomfort of the oral mucosa, then water alone may be used during tooth cleaning procedures.

Whilst a number of toothbrushing techniques have been described, a controlled gentle 'scrub' is recommended with emphasis placed on small movements and gentle pressure, together with an unhurried systematic approach to the cleaning of all surfaces.[19] Cleaning someone else's teeth is completely different from cleaning one's own teeth. Appropriate techniques are illustrated in Fig. 3.2. It is usually easier to provide assisted toothbrushing from behind the patient. The head should be cradled and supported by the arm and hand of the carer. If access from behind is not possible, or proves too uncomfortable for the patient, then an approach from the side should be adopted (Fig. 3.3). No more than two teeth should be cleaned at a time, and a systematic approach should be adopted, which ensures that all surfaces of all the teeth are included.

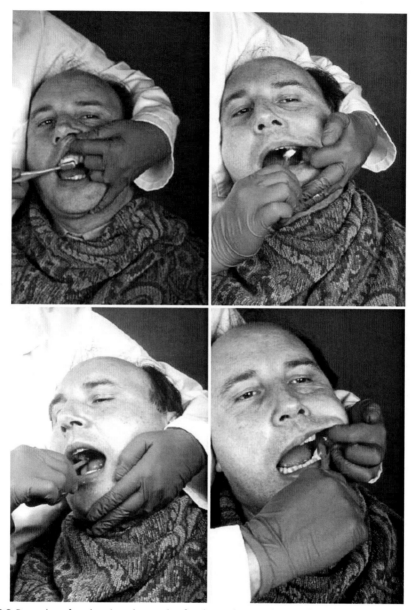

Fig. 3.2 Procedure for cleaning the teeth of a dependent patient with one operator.

(*Continued*)

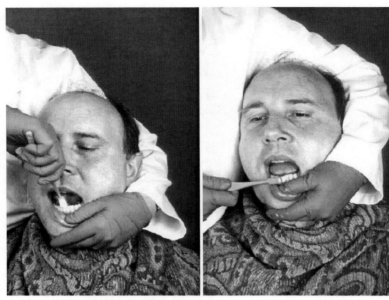

- Patient should be seated comfortably
- Clothes/pyjamas protected
- Patient's head must be well supported by operator
- The operator approaches from behind
- The lower jaw should be supported all times
- Soft tissues are carefully retracted
- Follow a systematic approach to ensure that all tooth surfaces are cleaned.

Fig. 3.2 Cont'd

Interdental cleaning

Interdental aids are designed to remove dental plaque from the areas between teeth that cannot be reached by a toothbrush. Ideally, some form of interdental cleaning should be used on a daily basis, though this may not be achievable for some seriously ill patients. The types of cleaning aids available include dental floss, dental tape, wood sticks and interdental brushes. It should be noted that some interdental cleaning aids may cause damage to the oral tissues if they are used inappropriately. Therefore, training on their use should be made available to staff.

Chemical plaque control

For some patients, mechanical plaque control is extremely difficult because of their level of debilitation. In such cases chemical plaque control may be considered for maintenance of oral hygiene.

Currently the most effective anti-plaque agent is chlorhexidine.[20] The chlorhexidine molecule has a positive charge at either end, and binds readily to negatively

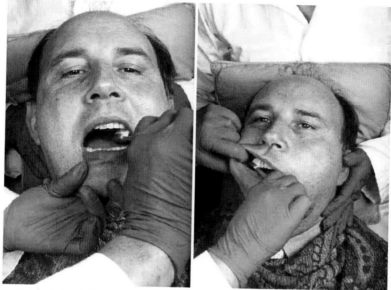

- Patient should be seated comfortably
- Clothes/pyjamas protected
- Patientís head is supported on a pillow or cushion
- Additional support for the neck is provided by the second operator
- The operator approaches from front or side
- The lower jaw should be supported at all times
- Soft tissues are carefully retracted
- Follow a systematic approach to ensure that all tooth surfaces are cleaned.

Fig. 3.3 Procedure for cleaning the teeth of a dependent patient with two operators.

charged sites on the enamel pellicle, mucosal cells and bacterial cell wall structures. Chlorhexidine is slowly released from surfaces, maintaining its antimicrobial activity, a property known as substantivity. In view of this property, there are no indications for using it more than twice daily.[21] Chlorhexidine exerts its antimicrobial effect by damaging the microbial cell membrane and precipitating the cell contents. It also inhibits microbial adherence.

It is important to realize that chlorhexidine will not remove established plaque. In clinical use therefore the mouth should be thoroughly cleaned, ideally by a dentist or dental hygienist, before the regular use of chlorhexidine to maintain a plaque-free environment. Chlorhexidine is used most commonly as a 0.2 per cent mouthwash (10 ml tow times a day), but it is also available as a 1 per cent gel and a 0.2 per cent spray.

The most common side-effect associated with long-term use of chlorhexidine is extrinsic staining of the teeth and the dorsal surface of the tongue. This does not happen in all patients, and is related to intake of tannin from beverages such as tea and coffee.[22] This staining of the teeth can be readily removed by a dental hygienist.

Other problems include the taste of the mouthwash, and the alcohol content, which may cause mucosal discomfort. Both of these drawbacks can be addressed by diluting the mouthwash with water (no more than 50 per cent).[23]

Denture care

Dentures become readily colonized with micro-organisms, acting as reservoirs of infection and predisposing to disorders such as denture stomatitis (see Chapter 6). It is, therefore, essential that a high level of denture hygiene is maintained.

Removal and insertion of complete dentures

Removal of dentures is a routine part of mouth care. If at all possible, patients should remove their own dentures. However, this may be difficult for debilitated patients, and care staff must become proficient at removal and insertion of both upper and lower dentures. This is a straightforward process if a few simple rules are followed. The technique to be adopted for denture removal is illustrated in Fig. 3.4. The lower denture should always be removed first to reduce any risk of aspiration. Reinsertion of dentures entails a reversal of the procedure (Fig. 3.5).

Removal and insertion of partial dentures

Partial dentures are often small and well-fitting, and are frequently mistaken for natural teeth. Most partial dentures are easy to remove and insert, but for some it is necessary to follow specific paths of insertion and removal. The patient and/or their family should be aware of the best way to insert and remove the partial denture, but if difficulties are encountered advice may be sought from the dental team. Small partial dentures are fragile and easily broken if force is used. If insertion and removal of the denture proves difficult and distressing for the patient, the denture should be left out of the mouth permanently, or until the patient is well enough to cooperate more fully.

Denture hygiene

Care of dentures must be carried out regularly and should be incorporated into a daily oral care routine, to ensure that it is done at least once per day (preferably at night). Cleaning a denture is not difficult and it should take no more than a few minutes to achieve a satisfactory result. All dentures, both partial and complete, must be cleaned outside the mouth and the soft tissues of the mouth cleaned separately. For those wearing partial dentures, especially those with wires or clasps to aid retention, the supporting teeth must be cleaned thoroughly.

Dentures, particularly acrylic dentures, are fragile and break easily if dropped. For this reason they should always be cleaned over a sink, or a bowl of water, so that if dropped they will not be damaged. The denture should be held under running water to remove loose food particles and other debris, then brushed thoroughly with a large toothbrush/denture brush, or a personal nailbrush, to dislodge any remaining plaque/debris from around the teeth and also the fitting surface of the denture. Commercial products are available for cleaning dentures, but household soap, or just

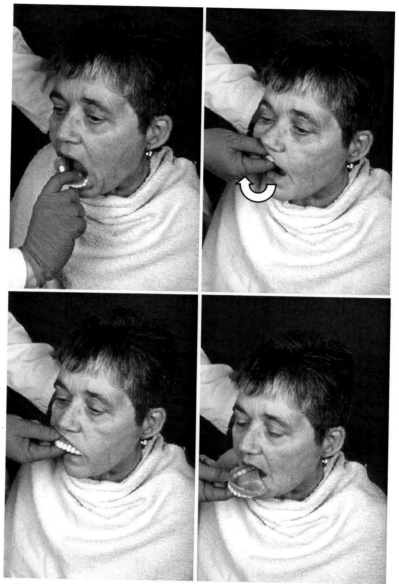

- The lower denture is removed first by grasping it firmly in the midline, lifting it upwards, and gently rotating it out of the mouth
- The upper denture is removed by grasping it firmly in the midline, breaking the seal with the palate, dropping it downwards, and gently rotating it out of the mouth. The seal is broken by tilting the denture forward while applying upward pressure on the front teeth, and supplying support to the back of the head.

Fig. 3.4 Procedure for removal of a complete denture.

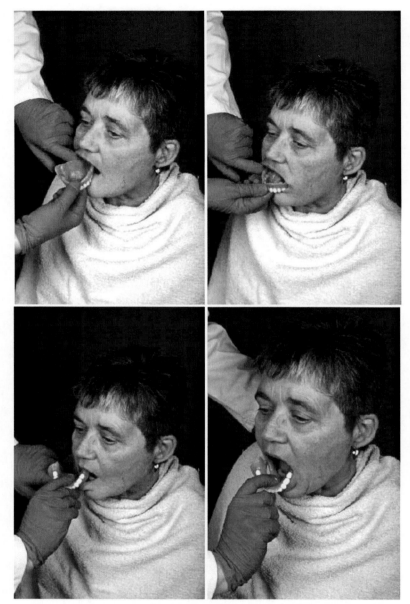

- The upper is inserted first by rotation, and seated firmly in place
- The lower denture is inserted by rotation, and seated firmly in place.

Fig. 3.5 Procedure for insertion of a complete denture.

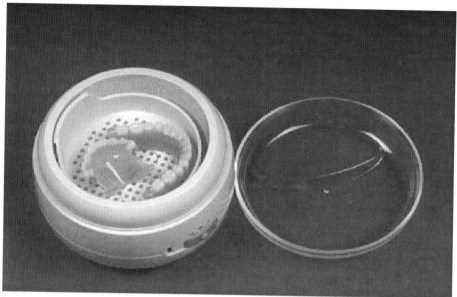

Fig. 3.6 An ultrasonic bath for denture cleaning.

water alone, is usually satisfactory. Ordinary toothpaste should not be used, because it is too abrasive and may damage the polished surface of the denture. The denture should be rinsed well before replacing it in the patient's mouth. Individual ultrasonic baths (Fig. 3.6) are available commercially to aid denture cleaning if resources permit.

Hard deposits of calculus (tartar) may form on the smooth surfaces of a denture as a result of calcium deposition from saliva. This may cause irritation or trauma, and should be removed professionally as soon as it is noticed.

In order to maintain a healthy oral mucosa, it is advisable to leave dentures out of the mouth at night. If patients are reluctant to leave their dentures out at night, they should be asked to remove them for at least an hour during the day. Plastic dentures should be soaked overnight in a dilute solution of sodium hypochlorite (1 part Milton® 1 per cent to 80 parts of water). This allows disinfection of the denture, and reduces the likelihood of a denture stomatitis. The denture should be rinsed well under running water before being returned to the patient's mouth. For those dentures with metal parts (cobalt-chrome dentures) sodium hypochlorite should not be used, as it can cause discolouration of the metal parts of the denture. Instead the denture should be soaked in chlorhexidine gluconate (0.2 per cent solution) to achieve disinfection. It should be noted that while commercially available products may be very effective in *cleaning* dentures, they might not be as effective in *disinfecting* dentures.

Distortion of the fitting surface of the denture can occur if the acrylic base dries out. Thus, some experts recommend storing dentures in water.[24] However, other experts

Table 3.3 Denture marking procedure

Time required	Approximately 10 minutes
Equipment required	Small piece of scourer pad Pencil or alcohol-based pen Clear varnish
Number of dentures marked at one time	Upper and lower dentures belonging to one individual only
Denture preparation	Clean and dry denture Select an area on the non-fitting surface of the denture, near the back that will not show when the denture is being worn Use the scourer to remove the surface polish from an area just large enough to take the person's name
Marking the denture	Neatly print the person's initial and surname Paint with a thin coat of the varnish Allow to dry Apply a second thin coat of varnish Allow to dry
Aftercare	Normal denture cleaning Check periodically to ensure the name remains legible (lasts ~ 6–12 months)

oppose storing dentures in water, particularly in dependent patients, because of the risk of promoting microbial growth.[25] The use of dilute sodium hypochlorite/chlorhexidine solutions should address both of these concerns.

For maximum patient comfort, dentures should be rinsed under running water after every meal, and the lining of the mouth checked for food debris before reinserting the dentures.

Dentures should be stored in a denture container clearly marked with the patient's name. Dentures themselves can also be marked with the patient's name. The decision to mark dentures depends on the individual circumstances. However, it is a good idea to mark the dentures of dependent patients, particularly if they are resident for any length of time in a care institution (hospital, hospice or nursing home). Denture marking is a relatively simple process (Table 3.3). Specific denture marking kits are available for purchase from dental supply companies.

Care of the oral mucosa

The oral mucosa should be cleaned 3–4 times per day, ideally after each meal. For those patients who are able, rinsing the mouth with water is adequate to remove food debris. For those who are unable to rinse, the mucosa should be cleaned mechanically with a water-moistened gauze or a foam stick (Fig. 3.7). If necessary, the tongue should be stabilized by holding with gauze and cleaned gently from back to front. It is important to remember to include the lips, to ensure that they remain free of debris.

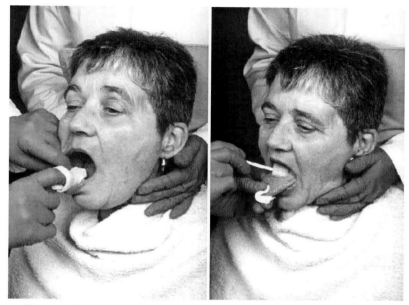

- The head is supported by a second operator
- A moistened piece of gauze wrapped around finger or a moistened foam swab is used to remove food and other debris from the oral mucosa
- The tongue should always be cleaned from back to front. (Cleaning the tongue is easier if the tongue is held/immobilized using a piece of gauze).

Fig. 3.7 Procedure for maintaining cleanliness of the oral mucosa.

An important aspect of care is the management of any coexistent xerostomia (see Chapter 9). It should be noted that oil-based products, such as petroleum jelly, are not recommended for lip protection, because of the risk of aspiration. Instead, water-based products, such as KY® jelly and Oralbalance® gel, should be used.

Oral care in the terminal phase

Oral care often takes prominence during the terminal phase of the illness. Indeed, oral care is a major component of 'care of the dying' pathways.[26] The provision of oral care is often determined by historical protocols, rather than by the needs of the patient. Moreover, there is very little evidence to support many of the interventions within these historical protocols.[14]

The philosophy of care in the terminal phase should be the maintenance of patient comfort. It is relatively easy to determine the merits of oral care in conscious patients. (Carers should always ask patients about their experiences of oral care.) However, it is much less easy to determine the merits of oral care in unconscious patients. If an intervention causes or appears to cause distress, then that intervention should be discontinued.

Some authors recommend 1–2 hourly oral care for certain groups of debilitated patients.[27] This is very obtrusive for patients (and families), and very time-consuming for the carers. Some patients require this frequency of care to maintain oral comfort but many require much less frequent care to maintain oral comfort. Thus, again, the frequency of oral care should be determined on an individual basis.

One of the most common problems amongst unconscious patients is the presence of a dry oral mucosa. The family and carers often perceive this as a source of discomfort and/or a sign of neglect. Oral protocols often recommend the regular application of water. However, this intervention is largely ineffective, since the water quickly evaporates. A more effective regimen involves the regular application of water-based products, such as KY® jelly and Oral Balance® gel. These products last longer, and so they need to be applied less often.

Oral care is often delegated to the family in the terminal phases.[28] Some family members relish this task, whilst others find it difficult/distressing. It is important, if appropriate, that families are given the opportunity to provide oral care. Equally, it is important that families are not coerced into providing oral care. Professional carers have a duty to provide adequate instructions, and on going support/supervision for this task.

Semiconscious/unconscious patients are at increased risk of aspiration. It is, therefore, essential that oral care regimens are adapted to minimise the risk of aspiration (use of non-foaming toothpastes; use of water-based lubricants).

References

1. DeConno F, Sbanotto A, Ripamonti C, Ventafridda V (2003). Mouth care. In D Doyle, G Hanks, N Cherny, K Calman (ed.) *Oxford Textbook of Palliative Medicine*, 3rd edn. Oxford: Oxford University Press.

2. Li X, Kolltveit KM, Tronstad L, Olsen I (2000). Systemic diseases caused by oral infection. *Clin Microbiol Rev* **13**: 547–58.

3. Eilers J, Berger AM, Petersen MC (1988). Development, testing, and application of the oral assessment guide. *Oncol Nurs Forum* **15**: 325–30.

4. Crosby C (1989). Method in mouth care. *Nurs Times* **85**: 38–41.

5. White R (2000). Nurse assessment of oral health: a review of practice and education. *Br J Nurs* **9**: 260–6.

6. Holmes S, Mountain E (1993). Assessment of oral status: evaluation of three oral assessment guides. *J Clin Nurs* **2**: 35–40.

7. Paunovich ED, Aubertin MA, Saunders MJ, Prange M (2000). The role of dentistry in palliative care of the head and neck cancer patient. *Texas Dent J* **117**: 36–45.

8. Mojon P, Rentsch A, Budtz-Jorgensen E, Baehni PC (1998). Effects of an oral health program on selected clinical parameters and salivary bacteria in a long-term care facility. *Eur J Oral Sci* **106**: 827–34.

9. Hunt M (1987). The process of translating research findings into nursing practice. *J Adv Nurs* **12**: 101–10.

10. Arvidson-Bufano UB, Blank LW, Yellowitz JA (1996). Nurses' oral health assessments of nursing home residents pre- and post-training: a pilot study. *Spec Care Dentist* **16**: 58–64.

11. Wardh I, Andersson L, Sorensen S (1997). Staff attitudes to oral health care. A comparative study of registered nurses, nursing assistants and home care aides. *Gerodontology* **14**: 28–32.

12. Rak OS, Warren K (1990). An assessment of the level of dental and mouthcare knowledge amongst nurses working with elderly patients. *Community Dent Health* **7**: 295–301.

13. Heanue M, Deacon SA, Deery C, Robinson PG, Walmsley AD, Worthington HV, *et al.* (2003). *Manual versus powered toothbrushing for oral health* (Cochrane Review). In The Cochrane Library, Issue 3. Oxford: Update Software.

14. Howarth H (1977). Mouth care procedures for the very ill. *Nurs Times* **73**: 354–5.

15. Harris MD (1980). Research: tools for mouth care. *Nurs Times* **76**: 340–2.

16. Pearson LS, Hutton JL (2002). A controlled trial to compare the ability of foam swabs and toothbrushes to remove dental plaque. *J Adv Nurs* **39**: 480–9.

17. Gaffar A (1998). Treating hypersensitivity with fluoride varnishes. *Compend Contin Educ Dent* **19**: 1088–94.

18. Griffiths J, Boyle S (1993). *Colour Guide to Holistic Oral Care: a practical approach*, p. 96. London: Mosby.

19. Levine RS (1985). The scientific basis of dental health education. A Health Education Council policy document. *Br Dent J* **158**: 223–6.

20. Jones CG (2000). Chlorhexidine: is it still the gold standard? *Periodontol* **15**: 55–62.

21. Loe H, Schiott CR (1970). The effect of mouthrinses and topical application of chlorhexidine on the development of dental plaque and gingivitis in man. *J Periodontal Res* **5**: 79–83.

22. Leard A, Addy M (1997). The propensity of different brands of tea and coffee to cause staining associated with chlorhexidine. *J Clin Periodontol* **24**: 115–18.

23. Axelsson P, Lindhe J (1987). Efficacy of mouthrinses in inhibiting dental plaque and gingivitis in man. *J Clin Periodontol* **14**: 205–12.

24. Jagger DC, Harrison A (1995). Denture cleansing – the best approach. *Br Dent J* **178**: 413–17.

25. DePaola LG, Minah GE (1983). Isolation of pathogenic microorganisms from dentures and denture-soaking containers of myelosuppressed cancer patients. *J Prosthet Dent* **49**: 20–4.

26. Ellershaw J, Ward C (2003). Care of the dying patient: the last hours or days of life. *BMJ* **326**: 30–4.

27. Anonymous (1996). *Managing Oral Care Problems Throughout the Cancer Illness Trajectory*, p. 9. London: The Macmillan Practice Development Unit.

28. Goodman M (2003). Symptom control in care of the dying. Section 3. In J Ellershaw, S Wilkinson (ed.) *Care of the Dying. A pathway to excellence*, pp. 55–7. Oxford: Oxford University Press.

Chapter 4

Domiciliary dental care

Angus Walls

Introduction

Domiciliary care is defined as 'a service that reaches out to care for those who cannot reach a service themselves'.[1] The term refers to care carried out in the patient's place of residence (e.g. home, hospice), rather than care carried out in a dental clinic. The first part of the chapter will discuss generic issues around the provision of domiciliary care, whilst the second part of the chapter will discuss the management of specific problems in the domiciliary setting.

Philosophy of care

The delivery of dental care is more complicated in any setting outside of the dental surgery. The plan of care that is developed for each patient must reflect both their oral health needs, and also what is practical in the circumstances in which the treatment will be delivered. Equally, the dentist must refrain from taking the easy option if this is to the detriment of the patient.

Procedures take longer in a domiciliary setting than they do in a surgery, and an individual's ability to sit or lie still for the length of time that would be required for a given task is a critical part of the treatment planning process. All treatment steps should be designed such that the dentist can very quickly stop the care they are providing if the patient's tolerance is becoming stretched.

Some cognisance also needs to be given to the patient's anticipated life span. An example for a patient with a limited life expectancy would be planning to produce a shortened dental arch, rather than struggling to maintain molar teeth.[2] The advantages of the shortened dental arch as a treatment philosophy are well established in the general population (maximal function from minimal intervention). However, one further benefit is apparent in those who rely on others for assistance with their oral healthcare: the teeth are more accessible at the front of the mouth than they are at the back of the mouth.

Type of care

Dental professionals are considered important members of the extended palliative care team.[3] Nevertheless, there is little data on their actual role within palliative care.

Walls *et al.* reported their experience of providing dental care over a 3-year period to a 15-bed hospice in the United Kingdom.[4] The main indications for referral were problems relating to dentures, rather than problems relating to teeth or oral mucosae (Table 4.1).

One of the reasons for the predominance of denture problems in this population is the high number of edentulous people in the general population. It should be noted, however, that this number is expected to decrease steadily over the next few decades.[5] The other reasons for the predominance of denture problems in this population are discussed below.

Provision of care

The provision of care for a patient depends on a number of factors: (a) the medical team identifying appropriate patients; (b) the medical team referring appropriate patients; and (c) the availability of domiciliary dental services. Oral healthcare pathways can be a useful adjunct in this setting. However, oral healthcare pathways need to be supported by relevant training for the medical team (and also for the carers). Dental professionals need to be involved in the development of oral healthcare pathways, and also in the provision of relevant training.

Setting

Ideally, dental care should be performed with the patient seated on a reclining chair. However, dental care can be performed with the patient lying on an ordinary bed. If the patient is lying on a bed, then the operator can sit to one side of the bed with the patient's head in their lap. A simple piece of board padded with bedding and placed under the patient to support their head is a great help in this situation.

Equipment

The equipment that the dentist, or dental hygienist, requires will depend on the treatment needs of the patient. A good source of light is vital. The most practical source of illumination is a battery-operated headlight (Fig. 4.1). There are now a number of sophisticated portable dental treatment units available that run from either mains electricity, or rechargeable batteries (Fig. 4.2). These units contain an E fitting dental motor, a small vacuum pump, and a 3 in 1 syringe. They can also be equipped with useful extras such as a curing light, and a piezon ultrasonic scaler. In addition to specialist dental equipment, the dental team will need to carry with them all the hand instruments and the materials that they are likely to require, some means of creating a clean working area and appropriate storage facilities for dirty instruments and materials.

Other issues

Oral/denture hygiene is an integral part of the domiciliary care process and is discussed in detail in Chapter 3.

Table 4.1 Dental problems encountered over a 3-year period in a hospice in the United Kingdom[4]

Complaint	Number of patients	Problem	Management
Loose dentures (difficulty eating)	26	Resorption of alveolar bone	Relining or replacement of denture
Loose dentures plus oral ulceration	12	Resorption of alveolar bone plus traumatic ulceration	Relining or replacement of denture
Loose dentures plus oral pain	10	Resorption of alveolar bone plus traumatic ulceration	Relining or replacement of denture
Nausea on inserting upper denture	4	Denture stimulating gag reflex	Adaptation (trimming) of denture
Oral discomfort/pain	5	3 – xerostomia	Management of xerostomia (see Chapter 9)
		2 – xerostomia plus dental caries	
Retention of food in cheek plus difficulty inserting denture	3	Facial paralysis	Adaptation (changing shape) of denture
Dental pain	2	Lost filling	Replacement of filling
'Rough' dentures	1	Dental calculus on denture	Removal of calculus (denture hygiene measures)

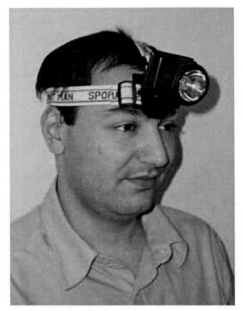

Fig. 4.1 Example of a portable light source.

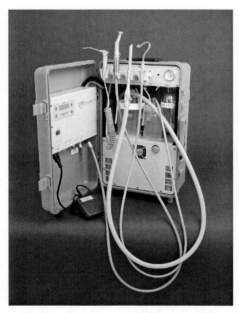

Fig. 4.2 Example of a portable dental treatment unit (Transport II Portable Electric Dental Unit, Aseptico Inc).

Table 4.2 Subjective dental problems in a hospice population[8]

Problem	Number affected by problem N = 22 (%)	Number bothered by problem N = 22 (%)
Food gets between teeth	17 (77)	8 (36)
Missing teeth	12 (55)	5 (23)
Sensitive teeth	10 (45)	2 (9)
Rough teeth	8 (36)	3 (14)
Dental cavities	7 (32)	1 (5)
Gum disease	6 (27)	2 (9)
Damaged fillings	6 (27)	1 (5)
Dental pains	4 (18)	1 (5)
Loose teeth	4 (18)	1 (5)
Dental infections	3 (14)	1 (5)

Dental problems

Dental problems are relatively common in palliative care patients.[6–8] The most common problems relate to dental caries, and to periodontal disease (Table 4.2).

The reported prevalence of active dental caries is 20–35 per cent.[7,8] Dental caries occurs in patients with advanced disease for two main reasons:

1. Xerostomia – Xerostomia is discussed in detail in Chapter 9.

2. Diet – One of the problems that patients with advanced disease often experience is a need to achieve high levels of calorific intake. Increased energy is most often achieved through the use of food supplements that are high in sugars, and that are continuously consumed during the day.

Caries needs to be actively managed with chemotherapeutic means in the early stages of disease (fluoride, chlorhexidine).[9] When necessary, the softened dentine should be removed, and the resultant defect restored. Caries removal can be achieved with rotary instruments ('drills'), or alternatively chemo-mechanically.[10] Chemo-mechanical removal involves the application of a compound, which softens the diseased part of the tooth, which permits removal of the diseased part of the tooth by hand instruments (rather than by rotary instruments). Chemo-mechanical removal has considerable advantages as anaesthetic may not be necessary, and the pattern of treatment is inherently gentle and careful. For caries on visible root surfaces, simple removal of softened dentine with hand instruments will often suffice.[11] The choice of restorative material is often dictated by the clinical situation: the material of choice is often a glass ionomer cement.

Theoretically, contemporary domiciliary equipment would allow for more advanced operative procedures, including endodontic care (root canal treatments) and full coronal restorations (crown replacements). One more advanced treatment option that is practical in a domiciliary setting is the use of adhesive bridgework to replace missing teeth, rather than the use of partial dentures. (Partial dentures are often poorly tolerated in this group of patients.)

Denture problems

Denture problems are very common in palliative care patients: the reported prevalence of subjective problems is 45–86 per cent[6–8] and of objective problems 57–83 per cent.[6–8] The most common problems relate to poor fitting of the dentures (Table 4.3). However, denture stomatitis and angular cheilitis are also very common (see Chapter 6). Thus, one study involving edentulous patients with advanced cancer found that 22 per cent had isolated denture stomatitis, 8 per cent had combined denture stomatitis and angular cheilitis, and 4 per cent had isolated angular cheilitis.[12]

The problems encountered are related to a number of factors:

- The age of the dentures – Aldred *et al.* reported that many patients had 'old' dentures (mean age – 16.5 years; range of ages – 4 months to 40 years).[7]
- The care of the dentures – Jobbins *et al.* reported that many (27 per cent) patients had unhygienic dentures.[8]
- The use of the dentures – a lot of patients (49–60 per cent) wear their dentures continuously, i.e. all day and all night.[7,8]
- Direct/indirect effects of the underlying disease.

It should be noted that data from the general population are very similar to these data from palliative care patients.[13,14]

Denture stability depends on a number of factors, particularly the quality of fit between the denture and the underlying bony ridge (consisting of mucosa, alveolar bone and basal bone). Alveolar bone progressively resorbs following tooth extraction.

Table 4.3 Subjective denture problems in a hospice population[8]

Problem	Number affected by problem *N*=14 (%)	Number bothered by problem *N*=14 (%)
Food gets under denture	12 (86)	7 (50)
Loose denture	10 (71)	8 (57)
Uncomfortable denture	8 (57)	7 (50)
Mucosal ulceration (denture-related)	6 (43)	6 (43)
Rough denture	4 (29)	3 (21)

The rate and extent of resorption is very variable. However, the result of resorption is that the there is a gradual reduction in the height and width of the bony ridge. The change in shape of the bony ridge has two major consequences:

1. A decrease in the quality of fit over much of the ridge, which may result in the development of denture instability;

2. An increase in the mechanical stress over the remaining points of contact, which may result in the development of mucosal ulceration and/or mucosal inflammation (leading to development of a denture granuloma/denture-induced hyperplasia). Figure 4.3 demonstrates a denture granuloma/denture-induced hyperplasia.

Patients and carers often associate the development of denture instability with weight loss. It is unlikely that weight loss has a significant effect on alveolar resorption, i.e. weight loss is not a major factor in the development of denture instability.[4]

Patients compensate for poorly fitting dentures by the use of habitual movements of the tongue, lips and cheeks. One of the consequences of advanced disease is that the patient will leave their dentures out of their mouth for long periods of time. This, in turn, will result in the patient losing their habituation to the prosthesis, and the oral juggling skills that they subconsciously rely on to stabilize their dentures will be forgotten. The dentures will then feel loose.

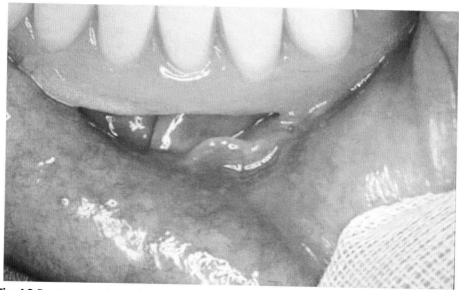

Fig. 4.3 Denture granuloma/denture-induced hyperplasia. Reproduced with permission from MP Sweeney and J Bagg (1997), *Making Sense of the Mouth*. Partnership in Oral Care, Glasgow. (See also Plate 6 at the centre of this book.)

The short-term solution to this problem is to use a chair side reline material. The options are a temporary soft lining, or a self-curing buteryl methacrylate product. The former is probably the better option. This approach re-establishes the adaptation of the denture base to the alveolar mucosa. It is, however, a short-term solution as there are problems with temporary soft lining materials becoming hard, and harbouring both bacteria and *Candida* species. Dentures with a soft lining should be cleaned, but not soaked, in chlorhexidine.

The definitive solution is simply to remake the prosthesis. The optimal approach for this is to use a denture copying technique.[15] This does allow some modification to the fit of the prosthesis, whilst retaining as much as possible the polished surface shape so that the new prosthesis appears to be familiar to the patient. It is highly likely that there will be significant technical problems with the dentures, for example inadequate lip support or occlusal errors. However, it is recommended that the emphasis be placed on producing a functionally good replacement, rather than a technically perfect replacement.

Denture stability also depends on the integrity of a salivary film between the denture and the mucosa. Thus, patients with xerostomia often have some difficulty in retaining their dentures. Moreover, patients with xerostomia are at increased risk of denture discomfort, and denture-related ulceration, because of the condition of the mucosa. Treatment of the xerostomia, as well as adaptation of the denture, may help to overcome these problems. (Xerostomia is discussed in detail in Chapter 9).

References

1. Fiske J, Lewis D (2000). British Society for Disability and Oral Health Working Group. The development of standards for domiciliary dental care services: guidelines and recommendations. BSDH.

2. Allen PF, Witter DJ, Wilson NH (1995). The role of the shortened dental arch concept in the management of reduced dentitions. *Br Dent J* **179**: 355–7.

3. Cummings I (1998). The interdisciplinary team. In D Doyle, GWC Hanks, N MacDonald (ed.) *Oxford Textbook of Palliative Medicine*, 2nd edn, p. 21. Oxford: Oxford University Press.

4. Walls AW, Murray ID (1993). Dental care of patients in a hospice. *Palliat Med* **7**: 313–21.

5. Steele JG, Treasure E, Pitts NB, Morris J, Bradnock G (2000). Total tooth loss in the United Kingdom in 1998 and implications for the future. *Br Dent J* **189**: 598–603.

6. Gordon SR, Berkey DB, Call RL (1985). Dental need among hospice patients in Colorado: a pilot study. *Gerodontics* **1**: 125–9.

7. Aldred MJ, Addy M, Bagg J, Finlay I (1991). Oral health in the terminally ill: a cross-sectional pilot survey. *Spec Care Dentist* **11**: 59–62.

8. Jobbins J, Bagg J, Finlay IG, Addy M, Newcombe RG (1992). Oral and dental disease in terminally ill cancer patients. *BMJ* **304**: 1612.

9. Jones JA (1995). Root caries: prevention and chemotherapy. *Am J Dent* **8**: 352–7.

10. Fure S, Lingstrom P, Birkhed D (2000). Evaluation of Carisolv for the chemo-mechanical removal of primary root caries in vivo. *Caries Res* **34**: 275–80.

11. Cole BO, Welbury RR (2000). The atraumatic restorative treatment technique: does it have a place in everyday practice? *Dent Update* **27**: 118–23.

12. Davies ANT (2000). An investigation into the relationship between salivary gland hypofunction and oral health problems in patients with advanced cancer. Dissertation. King's College: University of London.

13. Todd JE, Lader D (1991). *Adult Dental Health 1988*. London: HMSO.

14. Manderson RD, Ettinger RL (1975). Dental status of the institutionalized elderly population of Edinburgh. *Community Dent Oral Epidemiol* **3**: 100–7.

15. Davis DM, Watson RM (1993). A retrospective study comparing duplication and conventionally made complete dentures for a group of elderly people. *Br Dent J* **175**: 57–60.

Useful websites

British Society for Disability and Oral Health
http//:www.bsdh.org.uk

Chapter 5

Oral infections – an introduction

Susan Brailsford and David Beighton

Introduction

The oral cavity supports the growth of a diverse range of microflora (Table 5.1).[1] In excess of 500 different taxa have been isolated from the mouth using both conventional methods (culture techniques), and molecular methods (DNA sequencing).[2,3] The role of most of these taxa in health and disease has not been established. However, certain organisms, based on cultural studies, are recognized pathogens.

Colonization of the mouth

The oral cavity is sterile at birth, but within a few hours it becomes colonized by extraneous bacteria. The eruption of the teeth leads to changes in the oral microflora. For example, *Streptococcus mutans*, the organism classically associated with dental caries, is not detected prior to eruption of the teeth.[4]

After the eruption of the teeth, the oral microflora remains relatively stable, although the frequency of isolation of *Staphylococcus* species and *Candida* species (Figure 5.1) increases with age. This phenomenon of a stable microflora, within a changeable environment, has been termed 'microbial homeostasis'.[5]

The diversity of oral microflora is due to the variety of colonization sites. In general, the oral cavity is aerobic, and has a neutral pH. However, the gingival crevice is more anaerobic, and has an alkaline pH (7.5–8.5). The conditions within the gingival crevice favour the growth of certain periodontal pathogens (e.g. *Prevotella* species).

The teeth, the gingival crevice, and the dorsum of the tongue are invariably covered with a biofilm (layer of micro-organisms). However, other parts of the oral mucosa (buccal mucosa, floor of mouth, palate) are rarely covered with a biofilm, because of the rapid rate of epithelial cell turnover/desquamation within the oral mucosa.

Accumulation of micro-organisms within a biofilm allows them to survive by reducing their chance of removal by mechanical forces, and also by providing some protection from host defence mechanisms and exogenous antimicrobial agents.[6] It should be noted that within a biofilm there are areas with differing microenvironments, which encourage the proliferation of differing micro-organisms.[7]

In the following paragraphs, there is a simplified explanation of the development of dental plaque, which is defined as 'the community of micro-organisms found on the

Table 5.1 Commonly isolated oral micro-organisms[1]

Group	Genus
Gram-positive cocci Aerobic or facultative[†]	*Streptococcus* *Staphylococcus* *Enterococcus* *Micrococcus*
Gram-positive cocci Obligate anaerobes[††]	*Peptostreptococcus* *Peptococcus*
Gram-positive rods Aerobic or facultative	*Actinomyces* *Lactobacillus* *Corynebacterium* *Arachnia* *Rothia*
Gram-positive rods Obligate anaerobes	*Eubacterium* *Propionibacterium* *Bifidobacterium* *Bacillus* *Clostridium*
Gram-negative cocci Aerobic or facultative	*Neisseria/Branhamella*
Gram-negative cocci Obligate anaerobes	*Veillonella*
Gram-negative rods Aerobic or facultative	*Campylobacter* *Eikonella* *Actinobacillus* *Capnocytophaga* *Haemophilus* *Simonsiella*
Gram-negative rods Obligate anaerobes	*Bacteroides* *Fusobacterium* *Porphyromonas* *Prevotella* *Leptotrichia* *Wolinella/Selenomas*
Other organisms	*Mycoplasma* *Candida* Spirochaetes Protozoa

[†] = prefers anaerobic conditions, but can tolerate aerobic conditions
[††] = needs anaerobic conditions (cannot tolerate aerobic conditions)

surface as a biofilm, embedded in a matrix of polymers of salivary and bacterial origin'.[8] Readers are encouraged to consult a dental textbook for a more detailed explanation of these processes.

Colonization of the teeth occurs within minutes of them being cleaned. The salivary pellicle, which covers the teeth, forms the basis for the supragingival/subgingival biofilms.

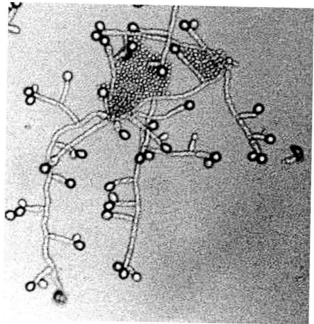

Fig. 5.1 *Candida albicans* (× 400 magnification). Courtesy of A. Davies.

The salivary pellicle consists of salivary glycoproteins, which have binding sites for bacteria ('adhesins').[9]

The main initial colonisers of the salivary pellicle are *Streptococci*, particularly *S. mitis*, *S. oralis*, and *S. salivarius*. These organisms are able to avoid host defences, and also to utilize salivary glycoproteins for growth. Other initial colonizers of the salivary pellicle are *Actinomyces*, particularly *A. naeslundii*.

The initial colonizers bind to the salivary glycoproteins, and other bacteria, using their surface structures (pili, fimbriae).[10] The initial period of bacterial adhesion/co-adhesion is followed by a period of bacterial growth. Saliva provides a source of nutrients for supragingival plaque, whilst gingival crevicular fluid provides a source of nutrients for subgingival plaque (see below).

Homeostatic mechanisms

A variety of different homeostatic mechanisms maintain the normal commensal flora, and prevent the development of oral infection (Table 5.2). Some of these mechanisms are non-specific (affect all micro-organisms), whilst other mechanisms are specific (affect only certain micro-organisms).

Oral mucosa

The oral mucosa forms a physical barrier to invading organisms.[11] Furthermore, the rapid turnover of the surface cells of the oral mucosa prevents the establishment of

Table 5.2 Homeostatic mechanisms within the oral cavity

Non-specific factors*	Oral mucosa
	Commensal flora
	Saliva
	Gingival crevicular fluid
	Complement
	Phagocytes
Specific factors*	Secretory IgA
	Serum IgM, IgG, IgA
	Lymphocytes

* Many of these factors are interrelated

a biofilm in many parts of the oral cavity. In addition, the surface layer of the oral mucosa is covered with a layer of saliva, and the deeper layers of the oral mucosa harbour immunoglobulins and lymphocytes (see below).

Oral infections occur in patients with oral mucosal damage. For example, patients receiving head and neck radiotherapy invariably develop oral mucositis, and frequently develop oral candidosis.[12] It should be noted that damage to the oral mucosa may lead not only to oral infections, but also to systemic infections.[13]

Commensal flora

Commensal organisms may utilize non-specific methods and/or specific methods to prevent colonization by pathogenic organisms. The non-specific methods involve competing with the pathogenic organisms for occupancy of the oral mucosa, and utilization of the oral nutrients ('competitive inhibition').[14] The specific methods involve actively suppressing the pathogenic organisms. For example, viridans streptococci can produce hydrogen peroxide, which inhibit periodontal pathogenic organisms.[15] Similarly, Gram-positive bacteria can produce bacteriocins (antibacterial factors), which inhibit certain pathogenic organisms.[16]

A number of factors can affect the commensal flora, including salivary dysfunction (see below), ingestion of antibiotics, and ingestion of high carbohydrate diet. For example, a high carbohydrate diet may cause a decrease in pH within the mouth, which favours proliferation of cariogenic micro-organisms, i.e. dental caries causing micro-organisms.[17]

Saliva

Saliva is very important for maintaining the normal commensal flora, and preventing the development of oral infections. Saliva has a number of different actions:

1. 'Flushing action' – the constant flow of saliva helps to prevent the adherence of micro-organisms.

2. Antimicrobial action – salivary gland secretions contain numerous antimicrobial factors, including secretory IgA (see below), mucin, lysozyme, lactoferrin, the salivary peroxidase system and histidine-rich polypeptides.[18] The mucins form a physical barrier to invading organisms; MG2 (a mucin) is also able to agglutinate certain invading organisms. The other salivary factors act in a variety of different ways. It should be noted that saliva is composed of salivary gland secretions, gingival crevicular fluid (see below), and various other components.[19]

3. Maintenance of pH – saliva maintains a neutral pH within the mouth. (The neutral pH within the mouth encourages the growth of commensal organisms, and discourages the growth of certain pathogenic organisms).

Salivary gland dysfunction is associated with significant changes in the oral microflora.[20] Furthermore, salivary gland dysfunction is associated with increased prevalence of certain oral infections (dental caries, oral candidosis),[21] and certain systemic infections (pneumonia).[22] Salivary gland dysfunction is discussed in detail in Chapter 9.

Gingival crevicular fluid

Gingival crevicular fluid is a serum transudate: the fluid passes from the systemic circulation, through the junctional epithelium of the gingiva, and into the gingival crevice/oral cavity. Gingival crevicular fluid contains a variety of antimicrobial agents, including complement, immunoglobulins (IgG, IgM, IgA), phagocytes (polymorphonuclear leucocytes, macrophages), and lymphocytes (B cells, T cells).[11] Moreover, the constant flow of gingival crevicular fluid helps to prevent the adhesion of micro-organisms.

Immune system

The innate/non-specific immune system within the mouth includes phagocytes (polymorphonuclear leucocytes, macrophages), and complement.[23] Phagocytes engulf and destroy a variety of different pathogens. They are derived from the blood, and enter the oral cavity in the gingival crevicular fluid. Complement has a number of functions including lysing/destroying Gram-negative bacteria, enhancing the action of phagocytes ('opsonization'), and promoting the migration of lymphocytes. Complement is derived from the blood, and also enters the oral cavity in the gingival crevicular fluid.

The acquired/specific immune system within the mouth consists of immunoglobulins (antibodies), and cell-mediated immunity (T cells).[11] The immunoglobulins include secretory IgA, and serum IgG, IgM and IgA. Secretory IgA is derived from lymphoid tissue within the salivary glands, and reaches the oral cavity in the saliva. Secretory IgA acts by preventing microbial adherence to host surfaces.[1] Serum IgG, IgM and IgA are derived from systemic lymphoid tissue, and reach the oral cavity in the gingival crevicular fluid. The serum immunoglobulins act in a number of ways – preventing microbial adherence to host surfaces, inhibiting microbial metabolism, or promoting microbial phagocytosis. T cells occur in a variety of different forms, which have a variety of different roles – stimulating B cells (TH2/T helper cells), and killing infected cells (TC/cytotoxic T cells).

Immunodeficiency is associated with changes in the oral microflora, and an increased prevalence of certain oral infections.[24] The pattern of oral infection is influenced somewhat by the nature of the immunodeficiency. For example, HIV infection/AIDS, which is characterized by a reduction in CD4+ cells (T cells), is associated with oral candidosis, periodontal disease, and oral hairy leukoplakia.[25] The development of these oral infections is strongly correlated with the CD4+ cell count (and the viral load).[26] HIV infection/AIDS is discussed in detail in Chapter 12.

References

1. Marcotte H, Lavoie MC (1998). Oral microbial ecology and the role of salivary immunoglobulin A. *Microbiol Mol Biol Rev* **62**: 71–109.
2. Hardie JM, Whiley RA (1999). Plaque microbiology of crown caries. In HH Newman, M Wilson (ed.) *Dental Plaque Revisited – Oral Biofilms in Health and Disease*, pp. 283–94. Cardiff: BioLine Publications.
3. Wade W (2002). Unculturable bacteria – the uncharacterized organisms that cause oral infections. *J R Soc Med* **95**: 81–3.
4. Kononen E, Jousimies-Somer H, Bryk A, Kilp T, Kilian M (2002). Establishment of streptococci in the upper respiratory tract: longitudinal changes in the mouth and nasopharynx up to 2 years of age. *J Med Microbiol* **51**: 723–30.
5. Alexander M (1971). Biochemical ecology of microorganisms. *Annu Rev Microbiol* **25**: 361–92.
6. Bowden GH (1999). Oral Biofilm an archive of past events? In HH Newman, M Wilson (ed.) *Dental Plaque Revisited – Oral Biofilms in Health and Disease*, pp. 211–35. Cardiff: BioLine Publications.
7. Vroom JM, De Grauw KJ, Gerritsen HC, Bradshaw DJ, Marsh PD, Watson GK *et al.* (1999). Depth penetration and detection of pH gradients in biofilms by two-photon excitation microscopy. *Appl Environ Microbiol* **65**: 3502–11.
8. Marsh P, Martin MV (1999). *Oral Microbiology*, 4th edn. Oxford: Wright.
9. Liljemark WF, Bloomquist C (1996). Human oral microbial ecology and dental caries and periodontal diseases. *Crit Rev Oral Biol Med* **7**: 180–98.
10. Kolenbrander PE (2000). Oral microbial communities: biofilms, interactions, and genetic systems. *Annu Rev Microbiol* **54**: 413–37.
11. Bagg J, MacFarlane TW, Poxton IR, Miller CH, Smith AJ (1999). *Essentials of Microbiology for Dental Students*. Oxford: Oxford University Press.
12. Redding SW, Zellars RC, Kirkpatrick WR, McAtee RK, Caceres MA, Fothergill AW *et al.* (1999). Epidemiology of oropharyngeal *Candida* colonization and infection in patients receiving radiation for head and neck cancer. *J Clin Microbiol* **37**: 3896–900.
13. Meurman JH, Pyrhonen S, Teerenhovi L, Linqvist C (1997). Oral sources of septicaemia in patients with malignancies. *Oral Oncol* **33**: 389–97.
14. Marsh PD (1994). Microbial ecology of dental plaque and its significance in health and disease. *Adv Dent Res* **8**: 263–71.
15. Hillman JD, Socransky SS, Shivers M (1985). The relationships between streptococcal species and periodontopathic bacteria in human dental plaque. *Arch Oral Biol* **30**: 791–5.

16. Balakrishnan M, Simmonds RS, Tagg JR (2001). Diverse activity spectra of bacteriocin-like inhibitory substances having activity against mutans streptococci. *Caries Res* **35**: 75–80.

17. Marsh PD (2003). Are dental diseases examples of ecological catastrophes? *Microbiology* **149**: 279–94.

18. Amerongen AV, Veerman EC (2002). Saliva – the defender of the oral cavity. *Oral Dis* **8**: 12–22.

19. Anonymous (1992). Saliva: Its role in health and disease. FDI Working Group 10 of the Commission on Oral Health, Research and Epidemiology (CORE). *Int Dent J* **42**, Suppl. 2: 291–304.

20. Almstahl A, Wikstrom M (1999). Oral microflora in subjects with reduced salivary secretion. *J Dent Res* **78**: 1410–16.

21. Sreebny LM (1996). Xerostomia: diagnosis, management and clinical complications. In WM Edgar, DM O'Mullane (ed.) *Saliva and Oral Health*, 2nd edn, pp. 43–66. London: British Dental Association.

22. Palmer LB, Albulak K, Fields S, Filkin AM, Simon S, Smaldone GC (2001). Oral clearance and pathogenic oropharyngeal colonization in the elderly. *Am J Respir Crit Care Med* **164**: 464–8.

23. Smith DJ, Taubman MA (1992). Ontogeny of immunity to oral microbiota in humans. *Crit Rev Oral Biol Med* **3**: 109–33.

24. Atkinson JC, O'Connell A, Aframian D (2000). Oral manifestations of primary immunological diseases. *J Am Dent Assoc* **131**: 345–56.

25. Chapple IL, Hamburger J (2000). The significance of oral health in HIV disease. *Sex Transm Infect* **76**: 236–43.

26. Campo J, Del Romero J, Castilla J, Garcia S, Rodriguez C, Bascones A (2002). Oral candidiasis as a clinical marker related to viral load, CD4 lymphocyte count and CD4 lymphocyte percentage in HIV-infected patients. *J Oral Pathol Med* **31**: 5–10.

Chapter 6

Fungal infections

Ilora Finlay and Andrew Davies

Introduction

A variety of different fungi have been reported to cause oral infections.[1] However, *Candida* species are responsible for almost all oral fungal infections. *Candida* species belong to the class *Fungi Imperfecti*, the order *Moniliales*, and the family *Cryptococcaceae*. This chapter will confine itself to a discussion of infection caused by *Candida* and related species, i.e. oral candidosis.

Definitions

Oral yeast carriage refers to subclinical colonization of the mouth. In contrast, oral candidosis refers to clinical infection of the mouth. Oral yeast carriage is a prerequisite for oral candidosis.

Oral candidosis is synonymous with oral candidiasis. However, most authorities use the term oral candidosis, since the suffix -osis is usually applied to fungal infections, whilst the suffix -iasis is usually applied to parasitic infections.[2,3]

Epidemiology

Certain *Candida* species are considered to be commensal organisms within the oral cavity. Indeed, the median reported prevalence of oral yeast carriage in the general population is 34 per cent.[4] Various groups of patients have greater levels of oral colonization. For example, the median reported prevalence of oral yeast carriage in hospitalized patients is 55 per cent.[4]

Oral yeast carriage is very common in patients with advanced cancer (prevalence 47–87 per cent).[5] Similarly, oral candidosis is very common in patients with advanced cancer: the prevalence varies between 8–83 per cent (see Table 1.3).[6–11]

Oral candidosis is also very common in patients with HIV infection/AIDS: the prevalence is up to 94 per cent.[12] It should be noted that the introduction of highly active anti-retroviral therapy (HAART) has led to a significant reduction in the prevalence of oral candidosis in patients with HIV infection/AIDS.[13]

Table 6.1 Aetiological factors for oral candidosis[14]

Yeast factors	Yeast species
Host factors	Immunological problems, e.g. cancer, HIV infection Endocrine problems, e.g. diabetes mellitus, hypothyroidism Nutritional problems, e.g. malnutrition, iron deficiency Iatrogenic factors*, e.g. antibiotics, corticosteroids
Intra-oral factors	Salivary gland dysfunction Oral mucosal damage, e.g. trauma, chemotherapy Presence of dental prosthesis (denture) Changes to commensal flora, e.g. antibiotics, salivary gland dysfunction

* See text for details

Aetiology

Candida species are relatively non-pathogenic organisms. Hence, oral candidosis usually occurs as a result of changes in host and/or intra-oral factors (Table 6.1).[14]

Yeast factors

Candida albicans (*C. albicans*) is the most common species isolated from the oral cavity, although increasingly other species are being isolated from the oral cavity e.g. *C. glabrata, C. dubliniensis, C. tropicalis, Saccharomyces cerevisiae.*[5,15]

Table 6.2 shows the primary yeasts isolated from the microbiological swabs of palliative care patients with oral candidosis.[16] The predominant organism was *C. albicans*: it was the principal yeast in 75 per cent of cases, although the sole pathogen in only 56 per cent of instances. In addition, *C. albicans* was isolated in another 8 per cent of cases. *C. glabrata* was the second most common organism: it was the principal yeast in 17 per cent of cases, although the sole pathogen in only 8 per cent of instances. *C. glabrata* was isolated in a further 17 per cent of cases.

Table 6.2 Primary yeast species isolated from microbiological swabs of palliative care patients with oral candidosis[16]

Yeast species*	Number of isolates N = 36
C. albicans	27**
C. glabrata	6
C. dubliniensis	1
C. tropicalis	1
S. cerevisiae 1	1

* C. = Candida; S. = Saccharomyces
** Seven patients had mixed growth

The main explanation for the increasing frequency of non – *C. albicans* species is the increasing use of antifungal drugs:[17] the use of antifungal drugs leads to the suppression of endogenous yeasts (i.e. *C. albicans*), which facilitates colonization by exogenous yeasts (i.e. non – *C. albicans* species). It should be noted, however, that there have also been significant developments in the identification of yeast species. For example, *C. dubliniensis* was only identified in 1995,[18] although it had been isolated as long ago as 1957.[19] (*C. dubliniensis* had been previously identified as either *C. albicans*, or *C. stellatoidea*.)[19]

The main consequence of the increasing frequency of non – *C. albicans* species is the increasing occurrence of antifungal drug resistance (see below).[15, 20] Drug resistance may be: (a) primary/intrinsic – this type of resistance develops de novo; or (b) secondary/acquired – this type of resistance only develops after exposure to the drug. *C. albicans* is inherently sensitive to the antifungal drugs, but it can develop secondary resistance to the azole group of drugs. Other *Candida* species have varying levels of innate sensitivity/resistance. For example, *C. glabrata* is inherently resistant to the azole group of drugs.[21] Similarly, *C. lusitaniae* is inherently resistant to amphotericin B.

Host factors

Immunological problems

Oral candidosis is very common in immunocompromised patients. The role of the immune system in preventing oral infections is discussed in detail in Chapter 5. Immunocompromised patients are at increased risk of developing secondary candidaemia/systemic candidosis (see below).

Iatrogenic factors

It is widely believed that systemic antibiotics cause oral candidosis. However, studies involving patients with advanced cancer have failed to identify such an association.[6,9,16] Moreover, a review of the literature concluded that 'the relationship between antibiotic therapy and candidosis is far from unequivocally proven'.[22] It is likely that systemic antibiotics contribute to, but do not cause, some cases of oral candidosis; the proposed mechanism being that the antibiotics suppress the commensal flora, which encourages the proliferation of yeasts.[14] There is a strong association between oral candidosis and the use of topical antibiotics.[23]

Similarly, it is widely believed that systemic corticosteroids cause oral candidosis. However, studies involving patients with advanced cancer have failed to identify such an association.[6,9,16] Moreover, a review of the literature concluded that 'the relationship between systemic steroid therapy and oral candidal carriage or infection is not clear'.[14] Again, it is likely that systemic corticosteroids contribute to, but do not cause, some cases of oral candidosis; the proposed mechanism being that the corticosteroids suppress the immune system, which encourages the proliferation/establishment of yeasts.[14] Nevertheless, other mechanisms may be important, such as increased salivary glucose levels.[14] There is a strong association between oral candidosis and the use of topical corticosteroids.[24]

It should be noted that Boggs *et al.* did report an association between oral candidosis and the combined use of systemic antibiotics and systemic corticosteroids in patients with advanced cancer.[6]

Other

Oral candidosis is associated with a poor performance status in patients with advanced cancer.[11]

Intra-oral factors

Salivary gland dysfunction

Oral candidosis is very common in patients with salivary gland dysfunction. The role of saliva in preventing oral infections is discussed in detail in Chapter 5.

Presence of dental prosthesis ('denture')

Oral candidosis is common in patients with a denture, particularly an upper denture. For example, a study from Denmark reported denture stomatitis in 65 per cent of elderly, community-living, denture-wearing people.[25]

Denture wearing can promote oral candidosis via a number of mechanisms.[26]:

1. Creation of a suitable environment for yeast proliferation – an artificial space is created between the denture and the mucosa. This space has a unique microenvironment, which encourages the proliferation of yeasts (i.e. relatively acidic, relatively anaerobic).

2. Protection of the yeasts adhered to the mucosa – the denture protects these yeasts from mechanical cleansing by the tongue, and chemical cleansing by saliva.

3. Protection of the yeasts adhered to the denture – *C. albicans* and *C. glabrata* can adhere to denture acrylic. The defects on the denture surface protect these yeasts from chemical cleansing by saliva.

4. Denture trauma – mucosal damage facilitates yeast colonisation/infection.

Clinical features

Oral candidosis can present in different clinical forms, sometimes several forms being found in one patient. Table 6.3 shows a recent classification system for oral candidosis,[27] whilst Tables 6.4 and 6.5 show the prevalence of these different types of oral candidosis in a palliative care population.[16]

Patients with oral candidosis may, or may not, have oral symptoms. Moreover, these symptoms may be due to the infection, or the underlying cause of the infection (e.g. salivary gland dysfunction). Indeed, many patients continue to have oral symptoms, even after they have been treated for oral candidosis.[28]

Table 6.3 Classification of oral candidosis[27]

Primary oral candidosis	Acute forms
	1 Pseudomembranous
	2 Erythematous
	Chronic forms
	1 Hyperplastic
	(a) nodular
	(b) plaque-like
	2 Pseudomembranous
	3 Erythematous
	Candida-associated lesions
	1 Denture stomatitis
	2 Angular cheilitis
	3 Median rhomboid glossitis
	Keratinized primary lesions superinfected with *Candida*
	1 Leukoplakia
	2 Lichen planus
	3 Lupus erythematosis
Secondary oral candidosis	Oral manifestations of systemic mucocutaneous candidosis

Pseudomembranous candidosis ("thrush")

Pseudomembranous candidosis is the most common type of oral candidosis. It is generally asymptomatic (see above). Pseudomembranous candidosis is characterized by the presence of off-white spots/plaques on the buccal mucosa, or elsewhere in the oral cavity (Fig. 6.1): the lesions can be easily removed.

Erythematous candidosis

Erythematous candidosis is relatively common. Patients often complain of localized discomfort/pain. Erythematous candidosis usually involves the tongue or the buccal mucosa, and presents as an area of inflamed (reddened) mucosa (Fig. 6.2).

Table 6.4 Prevalence of different types of oral candidosis in a palliative care population[16]

Type of oral candidosis	Number of subjects *N* = 120
Pseudomembranous	23
Erythematous	8
Denture stomatitis	15
Angular cheilitis	6

Table 6.5 Prevalence of different combinations of oral candidosis in a palliative care population[16]

Combinations of oral candidosis	Number of subjects $N = 120$
Pseudomembranous + denture stomatitis	5
Erythematous + denture stomatitis + angular cheilitis	2
Pseudomembranous + erythematous	1
Erythematous + denture stomatitis	1
Pseudomembranous + denture stomatitis + angular cheilitis	1
Pseudomembranous + erythematous + denture stomatitis + angular cheilitis	1

Denture stomatitis

Denture stomatitis is a very common type of oral candidosis in patients with dentures. It is generally asymptomatic, although some patients complain of palatal discomfort. Denture stomatitis is characterized by varying degrees of inflammation of the hard palate: the lesion may consist of patchy inflammation (Fig. 6.3), confluent inflammation (Fig. 2.1 (b)), and/or areas of hyperplasia. Denture stomatitis is often associated with angular cheilitis.

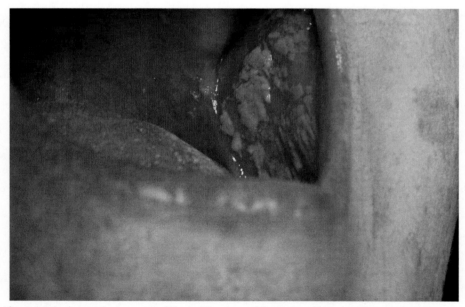

Fig. 6.1 Pseudomembranous candidosis. Courtesy of A. Davies. (See also Plate 7 at the centre of this book.)

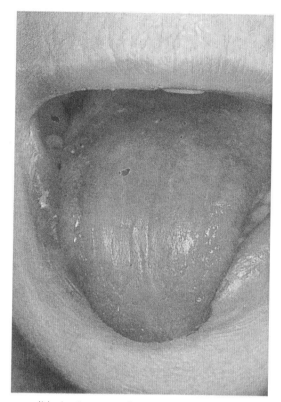

Fig. 6.2 Erythematous candidosis. Courtesy of A. Davies. (See also Plate 8 at the centre of this book.)

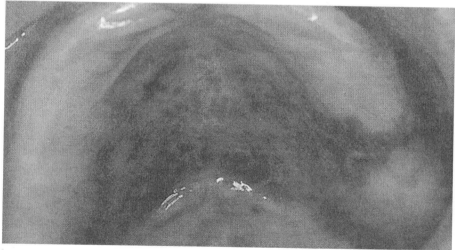

Fig. 6.3 Denture stomatitis. Courtesy of A. Davies. (See also Plate 9 at the centre of this book.)

Angular cheilitis

Angular cheilitis is relatively common, particularly in edentulous patients. Patients often complain of localized discomfort, and the lesions may 'weep' or bleed. Angular cheilitis invariably involves both angles of the mouth, and presents as cracking/inflammation of the mucosa and skin (Fig. 6.4). (The lesions may be covered with a crust/clot). Angular cheilitis may occur in isolation, or in combination with denture stomatitis.

Other types

The other types of oral candidosis are relatively uncommon. Figure 6.5 is an example of median rhomboid glossitis.

Oesophageal candidosis

Oesophageal candidosis is a frequent complication of oral candidosis.[29] The clinical features of oesophageal candidosis include odynophagia (pain on swallowing), and dysphagia (difficulty swallowing).

The diagnosis can be confirmed by performing an oesophagoscopy, or a barium swallow. The appearance on barium swallow is typical, with 'fluffy', punched-out lesions along the length of the oesophagus (Fig. 6.6).

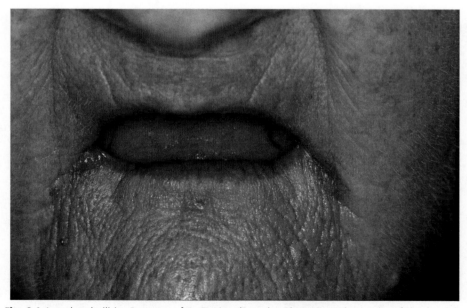

Fig. 6.4 Angular cheilitis. Courtesy of A. Davies. (See also Plate 10 at the centre of this book.)

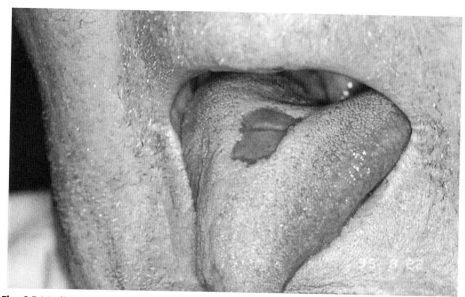

Fig. 6.5 Median rhomboid glossitis. Courtesy of J. Bagg. (See also Plate 11 at the centre of this book.)

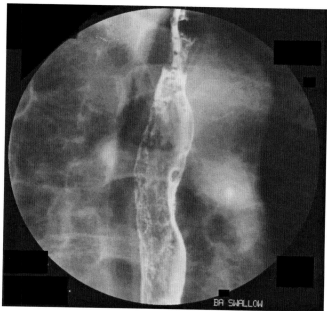

Fig. 6.6 Barium swallow showing oesophageal candidosis. Courtesy of I. Finlay.

Systemic candidosis

Candidaemia/systemic candidosis are recognised complications of oral candidosis. Immunocompromised patients (e.g. high dose chemotherapy patients) are at particular risk of developing these complications, as are other groups (e.g. intensive care patients).[30]

Candidaemia/systemic candidosis are associated with variety of different clinical features. Treatment is often delayed, because of difficulties in making the diagnosis. Indeed, in many instances, a definitive diagnosis cannot be made, and the patient is treated empirically. Treatment is often unsuccessful, because of a combination of delay in initiating treatment, the nature of the condition, and the nature of the underlying medical problem(s).

Investigations

A diagnosis of oral candidosis should be based on a combination of clinical features and microbiological investigations.[11]

The clinical features of oral candidosis are relatively non-specific. For example, white patches on the oral mucosa (akin to pseudomembranous candidosis) can also occur in bacterial infections.[31] Similarly, erythematous patches on the oral mucosa (akin to erythematous candidosis) can also occur in a number of other conditions, e.g. chemotherapy-induced mucositis.

As discussed above, it is common to isolate yeasts from the mouths of patients. Thus, a diagnosis of oral candidosis should only be made if there is heavy growth from targeted microbiological swabs. (A light growth would indicate oral yeast carriage, rather than oral candidosis.) Other microbiological tests are warranted if a patient suffers from persistent/recurrent oral candidosis (e.g. species typing, sensitivity testing).

Management

The management of oral candidosis involves:

- ◆ Treatment of the infection
- ◆ Treatment of the cause of the infection
- ◆ Symptom management.

A variety of different topical and systemic treatments are available for treating oral candidosis (Tables 6.6 and 6.7).[32–36] Oral candidosis usually responds to topical treatments. A recent Cochrane systematic review concluded that there was no difference in the results in studies comparing topical and systemic treatments.[37] Nevertheless, oral candidosis is often treated with systemic treatments.

The choice of treatment (topical/systemic product; polyene/azole drug) depends on a number of factors:

1. Extent of disease – topical agents are appropriate for treating localized disease, whilst systemic agents are more appropriate for treating multifocal/generalized disease.

Table 6.6 Topical antifungal agents available to treat oral candidosis in the United Kingdom[32]

Drug group	Drug	Recommended regimen	Side-effects	Comments
Polyene group	Amphotericin	1 lozenge (10 mg) qds 1 ml suspension (100 mg) qds 10–15 day course: continue drug for 48 hr after lesions resolved Increase dose in severe infections	Uncommon	Local action – drug needs to be kept in contact with lesions Resistance uncommon
	Nystatin	1 lozenge (100,000 U) qds 1 ml suspension (100,000 U) qds 7 day course: continue drug for 48 hours after lesions resolved Increase dose in immunosuppressed	Oral irritation/ sensitization Nausea	Local action – drug needs to be kept in contact with lesions Chlorhexidine may inactivate nystatin[33] – it is advisable not to use chlorhexidine immediately before/after using nystatin Resistance uncommon
Azole group (imidazole)	Miconazole	Apply appropriate amount of gel qds Continue drug for 48 hours after lesions resolved	Nausea and vomiting	Local and systemic action – drug needs to be kept in contact with lesions
Other agents	Chlorhexidine	See Chapter 3	See Chapter 3	Mainly used as an adjunctive agent[34] See above (nystatin)
	Gentian violet		Oral staining	Successfully used to treat oral candidosis in HIV patients[35]
	Tea tree oil		Oral irritation	Successfully used to treat oral candidosis in HIV patients[36]

Table 6.7 Systemic antifungal agents available to treat oral candidosis in the United Kingdom[32]

Drug group	Drug	Recommended regimen	Side-effects	Comments
Azole group (imidazole)	Ketoconazole	200 mg od (tablet) 14 day course	Nausea and vomiting Abdominal pain Headache Rashes Urticaria Pruritus	Not recommended for routine use in patients because of hepatotoxicity Monitor liver function Inhibits cytochrome P450 leading to certain drug interactions Resistance becoming a problem
Azole group (tiazoles)	Fluconazole	50 mg od (capsule/oral suspension) 7–14 day course Increase dose in severe infections	Nausea Abdominal pain Diarrhoea Flatulence Headache Rashes	Inhibits cytochrome P450 leading to certain drug interactions Resistance becoming a problem (Can cause liver damage)
	Itraconazole	100 mg od (capsule/oral liquid) 7–15 day course Increase dose in immunosuppressed	Nausea and vomiting Abdominal pain Dyspepsia Constipation Diarrhoea Headache Dizziness Menstrual problems	Not recommended for routine use in patients with/at risk of cardiac failure Capsule absorption dependent on low pH within stomach Inhibits cytochrome P450 leading to certain drug interactions Resistance becoming a problem (Can cause liver damage)

2. Drug resistance – resistance to the polyenes is uncommon, although resistance to the azoles is becoming increasingly common (see below).

3. Concordance/compliance – concordance with topical agents is worse than with systemic agents. (Many patients are unable to follow the treatment regimens of the topical agents – Table 6.6.)

4. Concomitant disease – the azoles have a number of relative/absolute contraindications, which may limit their usage.[32]

5. Concomitant drug treatment – the azoles have a number of drug interactions, which may limit their usage.[32]

6. Economic issues – the polyenes are generally cheaper than the azoles.[32]

7. Patient preference.

8. Availability of products/drugs.

It should be noted that the evidence for the effectiveness of individual antifungal drugs in treating cancer patients is relatively weak.[37] (The evidence of the effectiveness of individual antifungal drugs in treating patients with HIV infection/AIDS may be somewhat stronger.[38])

Many patients suffer with recurrent episodes of oral candidosis. The reason for this phenomenon is that although the infection is adequately treated, the underlying cause of the infection is not treated. For example, patients with oral candidosis secondary to salivary gland dysfunction will usually respond to antifungal drugs, but will often relapse on withdrawal of the antifungal drugs. However, studies have shown that treatment of salivary gland dysfunction significantly reduces the subsequent prevalence of oral candidosis.[39]

The successful management of denture stomatitis depends on a combination of antifungal drug treatment, and disinfection of the denture (see Chapter 3). Interestingly, denture stomatitis resolves if the denture is excluded from the mouth for a period of two weeks.[40] Similarly, the successful management of angular cheilitis in edentulous patients depends on a combination of topical antifungal drug treatment and disinfection of the denture. Furthermore, maintenance of denture hygiene is essential to prevent recurrence of these infections.

Prophylactic use of antifungal drugs

The mainstay of preventing oral candidosis rests with oral hygiene measures (see Chapter 3). The role of antifungal prophylaxis remains somewhat controversial.

A recent Cochrane systematic review concluded that there was 'strong' evidence that systemic drugs prevent the development of oral candidosis in patients receiving anti-cancer treatment (chemotherapy, radiotherapy).[41] The number needed to treat was calculated to be 9 (95 per cent confidence interval: 7–13). However, there was no evidence to support the use of topical drugs in this situation. Nevertheless, the authors were cautious about recommending the routine use of prophylactic antifungal drugs.

Similarly, another recent review concluded that there was 'good' evidence that fluconazole prevents the development of oropharyngeal candidosis in patients with HIV infection/AIDS.[38] However, there was 'insufficient' evidence to support the use of other antifungal drugs in this situation. In spite of such data, the United States Public Health Service/Infectious Diseases Society of America guidelines discourage the routine use of prophylactic antifungal drugs.[42] The main reason for the discouragement of antifungal drug use is the development of antifungal drug resistance (see below).

Resistance to antifungal drugs

Davies *et al.* have recently reported significant levels of azole resistance, but not polyene resistance, amongst oral yeasts isolated from palliative care patients in England.[20]: none of the isolates were resistant to nystatin, 2 per cent were resistant to amphotericin, 8 per cent were resistant to fluconazole, 22 per cent were resistant to itraconazole, and 7 per cent were resistant to ketoconazole. In most instances the resistant organisms were *C. albicans.* (The organisms that were resistant to amphotericin were non – *C. albicans* species). A number of the resistant isolates demonstrated cross-resistance for the azoles (i.e. were resistance to more than one of the azoles), and a number of the other isolates had relatively high minimum inhibitory concentrations for the azoles (i.e. were only sensitive to high doses of the azoles).

Similarly, Bagg *et al.* have recently reported significant levels of azole resistance amongst oral yeasts isolated from hospice patients in Scotland and Wales:[15] 23 per cent isolates were resistant to fluconazole, and 24 per cent were resistant to itraconazole. In most instances the resistant organisms were non – *C. albicans* species. Again, a number of resistant isolates demonstrated cross-resistance for the azoles, and a number of the other isolates had relatively high minimum inhibitory concentrations.

Antifungal drug resistance has also been reported to be a problem in patients with HIV infection/AIDS.[43]

The Standing Medical Advisory Committee Sub-Group on Antimicrobial Resistance (UK) concluded that 'Resistance to antimicrobial agents is a natural evolutionary response of microbes to antimicrobial exposure'.[44] Nevertheless, a review of the literature suggests that prudent use of antimicrobial drugs can limit the development of resistance, and that decreased use of antimicrobial drugs may reduce the levels of existing resistance.[44]

On the basis of the above, it is recommended that generally antifungal drugs, particularly azoles, should only be prescribed for microbiologically proven cases of oral candidosis. Furthermore, antifungal drug should be prescribed for short periods, since longer courses promote the development of resistance.[17] Similarly, antifungal drugs should be prescribed in high doses, since lower doses also promote the development of resistance.[17]

References

1. Odds FC (1997). Mycology in oral pathology. *Acta Stomatol Belg* **94**: 75–80.

2. Odds FC (1979). *Candida and Candidosis*. Leicester: Leicester University Press.

3. Samaranayake LP, MacFarlane TW (1990). *Oral Candidosis*. London: Wright.

4. MacFarlane TW (1990). Ecology and epidemiology of *Candida*. In LP Samaranayake, TW MacFarlane (ed.) *Oral Candidosis*, pp. 21–46. London: Wright.

5. Davies AN, Brailsford S, Broadley K, Beighton D (2002). Oral yeast carriage in patients with advanced carriage. *Oral Microbiol Immunol* **17**: 79–84.

6. Boggs DR, Williams AF, Howell A (1961). Thrush in malignant neoplastic disease. *Arch Intern Med* **107**: 354–60.

7. Rodu B, Griffin IL, Gockerman JP (1984). Oral candidiasis in cancer patients. *Southern Med J* **77**: 312–14.

8. Gordon SR, Berkey DB, Call RL (1985). Dental need among hospice patients in Colorado: a pilot study. *Gerodontics* **1**: 125–9.

9. Clarke JMG, Wilson JA, von Haacke NP, Milne LJR (1987). Oral candidiasis in terminal illness. *Health Bull (Edinb)* **45**: 268–71.

10. Aldred MJ, Addy M, Bagg J, Finlay I (1991). Oral health in the terminally ill: a cross-sectional pilot survey. *Spec Care Dentist* **11**: 59–62.

11. Davies AN, Brailsford S, Beighton D (2001). Corticosteroids and oral candidosis. *Palliat Med* **15**: 521.

12. Patton LL, Phelan JA, Ramos-Gomez FJ, Nittayananta W, Shiboski CH, Mbuguye TL (2002). Prevalence and classification of HIV-associated oral lesions. *Oral Dis* **8** Suppl 2: 98–109.

13. Schmidt-Westhausen AM, Priepke F, Bergmann FJ, Reichart PA (2000). Decline in the rate of oral opportunistic infections following introduction of highly active antiretroviral therapy. *J Oral Pathol Med* **29**: 336–41.

14. Samaranayake LP (1990). Host factors and oral candidosis. In LP Samaranayake, TW MacFarlane (ed.) *Oral Candidosis*, pp. 66–103. London: Wright.

15. Bagg J, Sweeney MP, Lewis MA, Jackson MS, Coleman D, Al MA *et al.* (2003). High prevalence of non-albicans yeasts and detection of antifungal resistance in the oral flora of patients with advanced cancer. *Palliat Med* **17**: 477–81.

16. Davies ANT (2000). An investigation into the relationship between salivary gland hypofunction and oral health problems in patients with advanced cancer. Dissertation. King's College: University of London.

17. White TC, Marr KA, Bowden RA (1998). Clinical, cellular, and molecular factors that contribute to antifungal drug resistance. *Clin Microbiol Rev* **11**: 382–402.

18. Sullivan DJ, Westerneng TJ, Haynes KA, Bennett DE, Coleman DC (1995). *Candida dubliniensis* sp. nov.: phenotypic and molecular characterization of a novel species associated with oral candidosis in HIV – infected individuals. *Microbiology* **141**: 1507–21.

19. Odds FC, van Nuffel L, Dams G (1998). Prevalence of *Candida dubliniensis* isolates in a yeast stock collection. *J Clin Microbiol* **36**: 2869–73.

20. Davies A, Brailsford S, Broadley K, Beighton D (2002). Resistance amongst yeasts isolated from the oral cavities of patients with advanced cancer. *Palliat Med* **16**: 527–31.

21. Fidel PL Jr, Vazquez JA, Sobel JD (1999). *Candida glabrata*: review of epidemiology, pathogenesis, and clinical disease with comparison to *C. albicans*. *Clin Microbiol Rev* **12**: 80–96.

22. Odds FC (1979). Factors that predispose the host to candidosis. In FC Odds (ed.) *Candida and Candidosis*, pp. 82–5. Leicester: Leicester University Press.

23. Lehner T, Ward RG (1970). Iatrogenic oral candidosis. *Br J Dermatol* **83**: 161–6.

24. Stead RJ, Cooke NJ (1989). Adverse effects of inhaled corticosteroids. *BMJ* **298**: 403–4.

25. Budtz-Jorgensen E, Stenderup A, Grabowski M (1975). An epidemiologic study of yeasts in elderly denture wearers. *Community Dent Oral Epidemiol* **3**: 115–19.

26. Budtz-Jorgensen E (1990). *Candida*-associated denture stomatitis and angular cheilitis. In LP Samaranayake, TW MacFarlane (ed.) *Oral Candidosis*, pp. 156–83. London: Wright.

27. Axell T, Samaranayake LP, Reichart PA, Olsen I (1997). A proposal for reclassification of oral candidosis. *Oral Surg Oral Med Oral Pathol* **84**: 111–12.

28. Finlay IG (1986). Oral symptoms and candida in the terminally ill. *BMJ* **292**: 592–3.

29. Samonis G, Skordilis P, Maraki S, Datseris G, Toloudis P, Chatzinikolaou I *et al.* (1998). Oropharyngeal candidiasis as a marker for esophageal candidiasis in patients with cancer. *Clin Infect Dis* **27**: 283–6.

30. Tortorano AM, Biraghi E, Astolfi A, Ossi C, Tejada M, Farina C *et al.* (2002) . European Confederation of Medical Mycology (ECMM) prospective survey of candidaemia: report from one Italian region. *J Hosp Infect* **51**: 297–304.

31. Tyldesley WR, Rotter E, Sells RA (1977). Bacterial thrush-like lesions of the mouth in renal transplant patients. *Lancet* **i**: 485–6.

32. Anonymous (2003). *British National Formulary* 46 (September 2003). London: British Medical Association and the Royal Pharmaceutical Society of Great Britain.

33. Barkvoll P, Attramadal A (1989). Effect of nystatin and chlorhexidine digluconate on *Candida albicans*. *Oral Surg Oral Med Oral Pathol* **67**: 279–81.

34. Ellepola AN, Samaranayake LP (2001). Adjunctive use of chlorhexidine in oral candidoses: a review. *Oral Dis* **7**: 11–17.

35. Nyst MJ, Perriens JH, Kimputu L, Lumbila M, Nelson AM, Piot P (1992). Gentian violet, ketoconazole and nystatin in oropharyngeal and esophageal candidiasis in Zairian AIDS patients. *Ann Soc Belg Med Trop* **72**: 45–52.

36. Vazquez JA, Zawawi AA (2002). Efficacy of alcohol-based and alcohol-free melaleuca oral solution for the treatment of fluconazole-refractory oropharyngeal candidiasis in patients with AIDS. *HIV Clin Trials* **3**: 379–85.

37. Clarkson JE, Worthington HV, Eden OB (2002). *Interventions for Treating Oral Candidiasis for Patients with Cancer Receiving Treatment* (Cochrane Review). In The Cochrane Library, Issue 4. Oxford: Update Software.

38. Patton LL, Bonito AJ, Shugars DA (2001). A systematic review of the effectiveness of antifungal drugs for the prevention and treatment of oropharyngeal candidiasis in HIV-positive patients. *Oral Surg Oral Med Oral Pathol Oral Radiol Endod* **92**: 170–9.

39. Rhodus NL, Liljemark W, Bloomquist C, Bereuter J (1998). *Candida albicans* levels in patients with Sjogren's syndrome before and after long-term use of pilocarpine hydrochloride: a pilot study. *Quintessence Int* **29**: 705–10.

40. Turrell AJ (1966). Aetiology of inflamed upper denture-bearing tissues. *Br Dent J* **120**: 542–6.

41. Worthington HV, Clarkson JE, Eden OB (2002). *Interventions for Preventing Oral Candidiasis for Patients with Cancer Receiving Treatment* (Cochrane Review). In The Cochrane Library, Issue 4. Oxford: Update Software.

42. Kaplan JE, Masur H, Holmes KK (2002). USPHS. Infectious Disease Society of America. Guidelines for preventing opportunistic infections among HIV-infected persons – 2002.

Recommendations of the U.S. Public Health Service and the Infectious Diseases Society of America. *MMWR Recomm Rep* **51** (RR–8): 1–52.

43. Denning DW, Baily GG, Hood SV (1997). Azole resistance in *Candida. Eur J Clin Microbiol Infect Dis* **16**: 261–80.

44. Standing Medical Advisory Committee Sub-Group on Antimicrobial Resistance (UK) (1998). *The Path of Least Resistance.* London: Department of Health.

Chapter 7

Bacterial infections

Jeremy Bagg

Introduction

Bacteria are responsible for dental caries and periodontal disease, two of the most common diseases of mankind. Bacteria are also involved in a range of other infections in the head and neck region, including dental abscesses, salivary gland infections and osteomyelitis.[1]

In recent years there has been an increasing focus on the association between oral infections and systemic health.[2] For example, there are significant concerns about the oral cavity as a reservoir for respiratory pathogens in elderly and debilitated patients.[3] Similarly, oral streptococci are a significant cause of bacteraemia in neutropenic patients with cancer, sometimes resulting in complications such as septicaemic shock, adult respiratory distress syndrome, and even death.[4]

Many bacterial infections require treatment with antibiotics. Antibiotics should be prescribed on the basis of the results of sensitivity testing. However, empirical treatment can be started prior to sensitivity testing, and definitive treatment started/continued after obtaining the results of sensitivity testing. Bacterial abscesses usually require drainage and may, or may not, require additional treatment with antibiotics. Clinicians should liase with the microbiology department about the most appropriate specimens to collect, and the most appropriate antibiotics to utilise. Furthermore, involvement of a dental surgeon is strongly recommended in the management of bacterial abscesses.

Dental caries

Dental caries is a chronic infection of enamel or dentine in which the microbial agents are members of the normal commensal flora.[5]

Epidemiology

Dental caries is common amongst palliative care patients. For example, the prevalence in hospice inpatients has been reported to range between 20–35 per cent.[6,7]

Aetiology

Lesions result from the demineralisation of enamel or dentine by acids produced by dental plaque micro-organisms as they metabolize dietary carbohydrates. Once the surface layer of enamel has been lost, the infection invariably progresses via dentine, with the pulp becoming firstly inflamed and later necrotic.

The main factors involved in the aetiology of dental caries are:

- Dental enamel – susceptibility to demineralisation by acid is probably related to many factors including the mineral and fluoride content, together with the structure of particular areas of enamel.

- Dental plaque – whilst there is continuing debate about the part played by some groups of bacteria in dental caries, there is substantial evidence of a role for *Streptococcus mutans*. *Lactobacillus* species are believed to be involved in the progression of carious lesions into the deeper regions of enamel and dentine.

- Diet – epidemiological studies have demonstrated clearly a direct relationship between dental caries and the intake of carbohydrate.[8] There is good evidence that the frequency of sugar intake, rather than the total sugar consumption, is of decisive importance in caries development. The most cariogenic sugar is sucrose, which acts as a substrate for the production of acids and extracellular polysaccharides. Extracellular polysaccharides are involved in the primary adherence of bacteria to surfaces and, more importantly, consolidate the attachment of bacterial cells to each other, thereby assisting the development of plaque.

- Saliva – saliva plays a number of important roles in preventing dental caries. The mechanical washing action of saliva is a very effective mechanism for removing food debris and unattached oral microorganisms from the mouth. Saliva has a high buffering capacity, which neutralizes acids produced by plaque bacteria. It is also supersaturated with calcium and phosphorus, which, together with fluoride, are important in the remineralization of early lesions.

Palliative care patients are at increased risk of developing dental caries, because of difficulty in maintaining oral hygiene, the presence of salivary gland dysfunction, and the presence of anorexia/weight loss (which results in the prescription of high energy/high calorie supplements).

Clinical features

The earliest clinical appearance of the disease is a well-demarcated chalky-white lesion in which the surface continuity of enamel is still intact (Fig. 7.1). This so-called 'white spot' lesion can heal/remineralize with the result that this stage of the disease is reversible. White spot lesions are asymptomatic.

As the lesion develops the surface becomes roughened and a cavity develops. If the lesion is untreated, micro-organisms extend the disease into dentine, and ultimately the pulp. Infections of the pulp are painful, and may progress to necrosis of the pulp. Figure 7.2 shows an example of advanced dental caries.

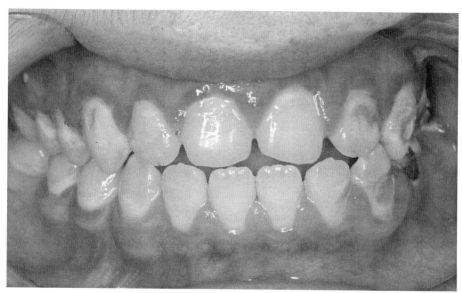

Fig. 7.1 Early dental caries ('white spot lesion'). Courtesy of G. Roberts. (See also Plate 12 at the centre of this book.)

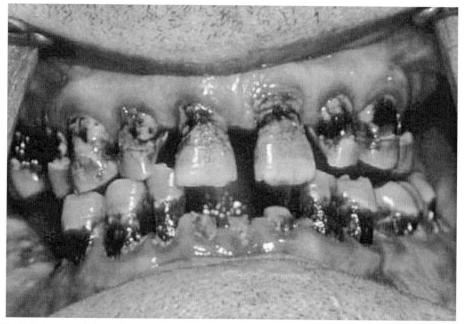

Fig. 7.2 Advanced dental caries. Courtesy of M Chambers. (See also Plate 13 at the centre of this book.)

Extension of dental caries commonly causes infection in the adjacent tissues, notably the periapical area, and orofacial soft tissues.[1] More rarely, infection may become established in the bones of the jaw to cause osteomyelitis.

Management

In the past, the general approach to treating dental caries was to remove diseased tissue and replace it with an inert restoration. The modern philosophy in dental caries management highlights the importance of active prevention, accurate early diagnosis, encouraging remineralization where appropriate, and minimal invasive techniques.

The most common approaches used in caries prevention are:

- Sugar substitutes – the use of artificial sweeteners is based on the premise that they cannot be absorbed and metabolized by plaque bacteria to produce acid. They may also reduce caries by stimulating salivary flow and encouraging remineralization. Sugar substitutes include those with a calorific value, for example the sugar alcohols and lycasin, and the non-nutritive sweeteners such as xylitol and saccharin. Evidence suggests that replacement of sucrose with sorbitol and xylitol may significantly decrease the incidence of dental caries.[9]

- Fluoride – fluoride can protect teeth from carious attack in several ways. Ingestion of fluoride, or its topical application, will result in conversion of enamel hydroxyapatite into fluorapatite, which is less soluble in acid. Fluoride also inhibits plaque metabolism.

- Mechanical cleaning – conventional toothbrushing with a fluoridated toothpaste is associated with an overall reduction in the incidence of caries. Other aids for plaque removal, for example interdental brushes, wood sticks and dental floss, may achieve some reduction in interdental caries, but there is less evidence for this.

- Antimicrobial agents – chlorhexidine is by far the most effective agent in controlling dental plaque formation.[10] At high concentrations the antiseptic is bactericidal by damaging cell walls. Chlorhexidine also binds to oral surfaces (especially teeth) and is then slowly released into saliva over many hours at bacteriostatic concentrations: chlorhexidine abolishes the activity of certain bacterial sugar transport systems, which reduces acid production in plaque. It is also possible that the presence of chlorhexidine on enamel surfaces and in saliva interferes with the adherence of plaque-forming bacteria, thus reducing the rate of plaque accumulation.

- Fissure sealants – these prevent caries in pits and fissures by blocking potential routes of infection by oral bacteria deep within the tooth.

The management of dental caries is discussed further in Chapter 4.

Dentoalveolar abscess

This common infection develops typically at the apices of the roots of teeth, following pulpal necrosis.[11]

Clinical features

The clinical presentation is dependent on the local anatomy, the pathogenicity of the infecting organisms, and the adequacy of treatment. If the abscess remains localized within the alveolar bone, the tooth will be very tender to pressure. Alternatively, the infection may burst through the alveolar bone and into the soft tissues. This may result in intra- or extra-oral swelling, or in potentially dangerous spread of infection through fascial planes.

Management

The essential element of treatment is to establish drainage of the pus. This can be achieved in several ways, depending on the clinical circumstances. If the tooth is expendable, then extraction will allow drainage. For teeth that are to be retained, drainage should be established through the root canal, and by incision of any residual fluctuant collection of pus.

Antimicrobial agents are not required in every case. They are useful as an initial approach to treat patients with gross facial swelling for whom drainage cannot be established immediately, and are useful adjuncts to drainage in patients who are febrile and/or immunocompromised. Amoxicillin is a suitable agent, whilst erythromycin is appropriate for those with penicillin hypersensitivity. Since many of these infections have an anaerobic component, metronidazole may also be used.

Periodontal disease

Periodontal disease in its widest sense includes all disorders of the supporting structures of the teeth, namely the gingiva, periodontal ligament and alveolar bone (Fig. 7.3). This may vary from inflammation of the gingiva alone, termed gingivitis, to the severe inflammation of the periodontal ligament, called periodontitis, in which there is destruction of alveolar bone and eventual tooth loss.

Epidemiology

Periodontal disease is common amongst palliative care patients. For example, the prevalence in hospice inpatients of 'active gingivitis' has been reported to be 36 per cent.[12]

Aetiology

Periodontal diseases are associated with a shift in the balance of the resident oral microflora.[5] The micro-organisms may produce disease directly by tissue invasion, or indirectly via bacterial toxins. The host response may be protective, for example phagocytosis of invading bacteria, or destructive, for example immune-complex activation of osteoclasts. Frequently it is a combination of both, and the interaction between these components determines the wide spectrum of disease that is seen clinically.

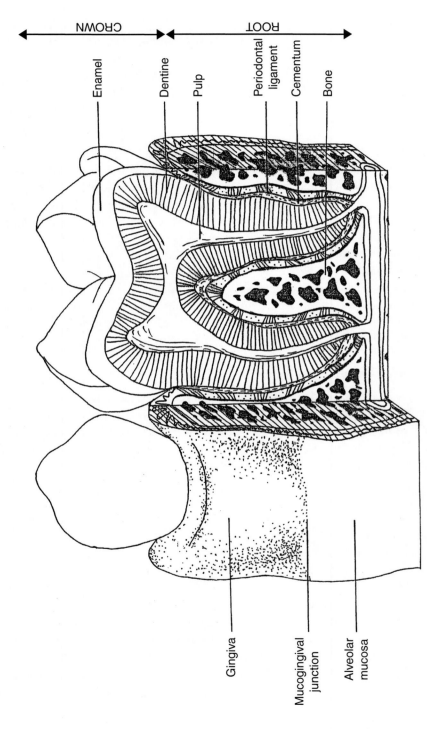

Fig. 7.3 Anatomy of gingiva/teeth. Courtesy of the Department of Anatomy, University of Bristol.

Several hypotheses have evolved to explain the part played by microorganisms in periodontal disease:

- The 'specific plaque hypothesis' – this suggests that only a small number of species are responsible for causing each type of periodontal disease. *Porphyromonas gingivalis, Prevotella intermedia, Bacteroides forsythus* and *Actinobacillus actinomycetemcomitans* are currently viewed as the mainstream periodontal pathogens.

- The 'non-specific plaque hypothesis' – this proposes that bacteria have collectively the total complement of virulence factors required to cause destruction of the periodontal tissues, and that some micro-organisms can substitute for others which are not present in the pathogenic consortia.

- The 'ecological plaque hypothesis' – this suggests that conditions within the periodontal pocket allow the overgrowth of certain organisms already present in low numbers, and that this shift in balance predisposes the site to disease. This theory may be viewed as a combination of the specific and non-specific plaque hypotheses.

Whichever hypothesis turns out to be correct, periodontitis clearly results from the activity of mixtures of interacting bacteria. All studies agree that there is a progressive change in the composition of the flora from health to gingivitis to periodontitis.

Some of the factors that may increase host susceptibility to infection include inadequate or unregulated host immune response, diabetes mellitus, stress and tobacco use.

Clinical features

The classification of periodontal diseases is a complex and contentious issue, addressed most recently by the American Academy of Periodontology.[13] A simplified classification will be employed in this chapter.

Gingivitis

There are several types of gingivitis. The most common of these is plaque-associated chronic marginal gingivitis, which is characterized by redness, gingival bleeding and oedema (Fig. 7.4).

Acute necrotizing ulcerative gingivitis is a specific form of gingivitis in which there is necrosis of the tips of the gingival papillae, spontaneous bleeding, pain and halitosis (Fig. 7.5).[14] In severely immunosuppressed patients, necrotizing ulcerative gingivitis can rapidly progress to a necrotizing ulcerative stomatitis, involving mucosa and bone.[15]

Among the immunocompromised, gingivitis often presents in clinically atypical forms. HIV-associated gingivitis is characterized by a band-like marginal erythema, usually accompanied by diffuse redness, which extends onto the vestibular mucosa (Fig. 16.4).[16]

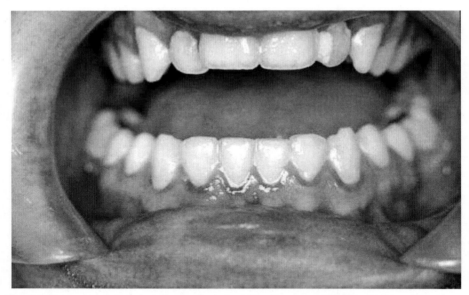

Fig. 7.4 Plaque-associated chronic marginal gingivitis. Courtesy of Prof David Wray. (See also Plate 14 at the centre of this book.)

Periodontitis

Gingivitis generally precedes periodontitis. The exact mechanism for the transition from gingivitis to periodontitis is unknown.

It can be subdivided clinically into several groups, the commonest of which is adult periodontitis.[17] Adult periodontitis may have its onset in adolescence and continue

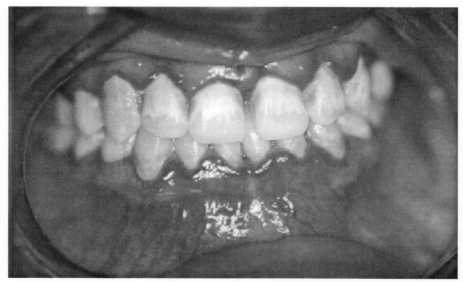

Fig. 7.5 Acute necrotizing ulcerative gingivitis. Courtesy of Dr Valli Meeks. (See also Plate 15 at the centre of this book.)

throughout the life of the individual, the severity increasing with age. It has been proposed that the disease occurs in short bursts of destruction, followed by periods of inactivity, these occurring randomly with respect to time and site within an individual.

In addition to gingival inflammation, adult periodontitis is characterised by destruction of alveolar bone and periodontal ligament (Fig. 7.6). As part of this process, periodontal pockets develop around the affected teeth.

Management

A summary of methods available for treating periodontal diseases has been published recently by the American Academy of Periodontology.[18] The main methods for treating periodontal diseases can be summarized as follows:

- ◆ Supragingival plaque control – see above.
- ◆ Scaling/root planing.
- ◆ Surgical therapy – surgery may be used to improve access for treatment, and to regenerate/reconstruct lost periodontal tissue.
- ◆ Consideration of adjunctive antimicrobial agents – antibiotics may be required for management of acute periodontal conditions, such as metronidazole for the treatment of acute ulcerative gingivitis, and penicillin for an acute periodontal abscess (see below). However, systemic antibiotics have no place in the routine treatment of chronic periodontitis. Locally delivered antibiotics (usually tetracycline or metronidazole) inserted into pockets, may occasionally have a role to play in the treatment of refractory periodontitis in the presence of adequate supragingival plaque control.

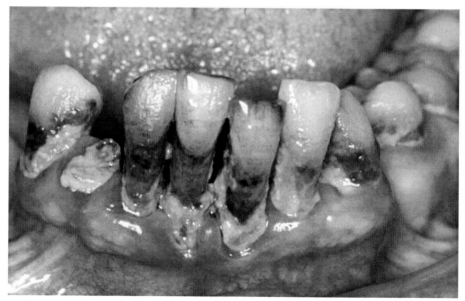

Fig. 7.6 Adult periodontitis. Courtesy of J Bagg. (See also Plate 16 at the centre of this book.)

Periodontal abscess

Periodontal abscesses usually occur in patients with established periodontal pockets.[19] Occlusion of the opening of the pocket prevents normal drainage, and results in an acute episode.

Clinical features

There is typically sudden onset of swelling, redness and tenderness of the gingiva. These abscesses frequently drain themselves along the root surface to the pocket opening, but if occlusion of the pocket is complete there may be local spread of infection with destruction of soft tissue and bone.

Management

Treatment options include extraction of the tooth, or drainage of the abscess followed by appropriate periodontal treatment. Antibiotics may be considered as an adjunct to treatment.

Oral mucosal infections

Bacterial infections of the oral mucosa are uncommon in developed countries, and are often manifestations of systemic diseases, for example gonorrhoea, syphilis, or tuberculosis. Such infections are seen more frequently in many developing countries.

Staphylococcal mucositis

Staphylococcus aureus has recently been incriminated as a cause of severe mucositis in some groups with systemic disease, including dependent (semi-comatose, dehydrated) elderly patients,[20] and patients with Crohn's disease.[21]

Clinical features

The clinical presentation starts with oral discomfort and mucosal erythema, progressing to widespread crusting and bleeding of the oral mucosa (Figs 7.7 and 7.8). There is a serious risk of aspiration of the infected fibrinous crust.

Management

Treatment involves careful removal of the fibrinous crust using a water-moistened gauze, followed by institution of regular oral hygiene measures (see Chapter 3). A course of an appropriate antibiotic (e.g. flucloxacillin for penicillin-tolerant patients) may hasten resolution, but is no substitute for ongoing regular oral hygiene measures.

Salivary gland infections

A number of factors are involved in the pathogenesis of salivary gland infections:

- ◆ Reduced salivary flow – oral bacteria are normally prevented from invading the salivary gland tissue by the natural flushing activity of saliva.

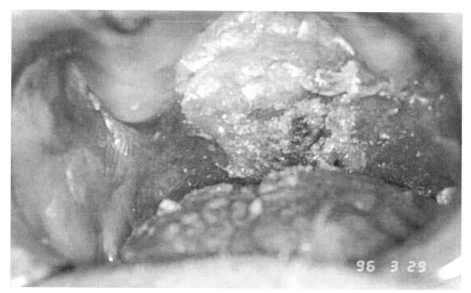

Fig. 7.7 Staphylococcal mucositis. Courtesy of MP Sweeney. (See also Plate 17 at the centre of this book.)

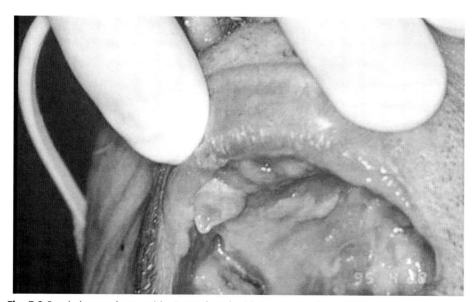

Fig. 7.8 Staphylococcal mucositis. Reproduced with permission from MP Sweeney and J Bagg (1997), *Making Sense of the Mouth*. Partnership in Oral Care, Glasgow. (See also Plate 18 at the centre of this book.)

- Salivary gland abnormalities (e.g. salivary calculi, strictures of ducts, dilatation of ducts).

Acute bacterial parotitis

The causative micro-organisms have not been well defined. *Staphylococcus aureus* and alpha-haemolytic *streptococci* have been most commonly reported, but *Haemophilus* species and anaerobes are also implicated.

Clinical features

Clinically there is a sudden onset of erythematous, firm swelling in the pre- and post-auricular areas, extending to the angle of the mandible. The swelling is associated with extreme local pain and tenderness. Milking of the parotid duct produces a thick, purulent discharge at the duct orifice (Fig. 7.9). Patients may be febrile.

Management

Treatment relies on appropriate antimicrobial therapy, ideally guided by the results of culture and sensitivity tests on a pus specimen.[22] Until such results are available, a penicillinase-resistant penicillin, for example flucloxacillin, should be administered. Erythromycin is suitable for patients with penicillin hypersensitivity. Increased fluid intake is important. In severe cases, antibiotic treatment may need to be supplemented with surgical drainage.

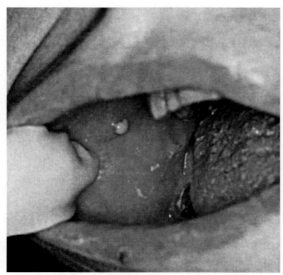

Fig. 7.9 Acute bacterial parotitis (pus draining from the parotid duct). Reproduced with permission from WR Tyldesley and A Field (1993), *Oral Medicine*, 4th edn, Oxford University Press, Oxford. (See also Plate 19 at the centre of this book.)

Following resolution of the acute infection, patients should be examined for factors which may have predisposed them to infection. This typically entails sialography, or a related imaging technique, to identify any correctable salivary gland abnormalities such as calculi or strictures. Sialography should never be performed during the acute infection.

Chronic bacterial parotitis

Some adults suffer recurrent episodes of parotitis. These are often a result of persistence of the aetiological agent (see above).

Clinical features

Unilateral or bilateral swelling of the parotid gland can occur, lasting from a few days to months. The clinical course is of intermittent exacerbations and remissions. This chronic, low-grade infection can functionally destroy the gland.

Management

Conservative therapy with antibiotics is recommended initially, but parotidectomy may be appropriate for long-term chronic parotitis.

Other salivary gland infections

Salivary gland infections usually affect the parotid glands, but may affect the other salivary glands, particularly the submandibular glands.

The salivary glands may also become infected in tuberculosis, and actinomycosis.[1]

References

1. Bagg J, MacFarlane TW, Poxton IR, Miller CH, Smith AJ (1999). *Essentials of Microbiology for Dental Students*. Oxford: Oxford University Press.
2. Li X, Kolltveit KM, Tronstad L, Olsen I (2000). Systemic diseases caused by oral infection. *Clin Microbiol Rev* **13**: 547–58.
3. Scannapieco FA (1999). Role of oral bacteria in respiratory infection. *J Periodontol* **70**: 793–802.
4. Marron A, Carratala J, Gonzalez-Barca E, Fernandez-Sevilla A, Alcaide F, Gudiol F (2000). Serious complications of bacteremia caused by Viridans streptococci in neutropenic patients with cancer. *Clin Infect Dis* **31**: 1126–30.
5. Marsh P, Martin MV (1999). *Oral Microbiology*, 4th edn. Oxford: Wright.
6. Aldred MJ, Addy M, Bagg J, Finlay I (1991). Oral health in the terminally ill: a cross-sectional pilot survey. *Spec Care Dentist* **11**: 59–62.
7. Jobbins J, Bagg J, Finlay IG, Addy M, Newcombe RG (1992). Oral and dental disease in terminally ill cancer patients. *BMJ* **304**: 1612.
8. Sheiham A (2001). Dietary effects on dental diseases. *Public Health Nutr* **4**: 569–91.
9. Hayes C (2001). The effect of non-cariogenic sweeteners on the prevention of dental caries: a review of the evidence. *J Dent Educ* **65**: 1106–9.
10. Jones CG (1997). Chlorhexidine: is it still the gold standard? *Periodontol 2000* **15**: 55–62.

11. Lewis MA, MacFarlane TW, McGowan DA (1990). A microbiological and clinical review of the acute dentoalveolar abscess. *Br J Oral Maxillofac Surg* **28**: 359–66.

12. Gordon SR, Berkey DB, Call RL (1985). Dental need among hospice patients in Colorado: a pilot study. *Gerodontics* **1**: 125–9.

13. Armitage GC (1999). Development of a classification system for periodontal diseases and conditions. *Ann Periodontol* **4**: 1–6.

14. Rowland RW (1999). Necrotizing ulcerative gingivitis. *Ann Periodontol* **4**: 65–73.

15. Patton LL, McKaig R (1998). Rapid progression of bone loss in HIV-associated necrotizing ulcerative stomatitis. *J Periodontol* **69**: 710–16.

16. Holmstrup P, Westergaard J (1998). HIV infection and periodontal diseases. *Periodontol 2000* **18**: 37–46.

17. Flemmig TF (1999). Periodontitis. *Ann Periodontol* **4**: 32–8.

18. Research, Science and Therapy Committee of the American Academy of Periodontology (2001). Treatment of plaque-induced gingivitis, chronic periodontitis, and other clinical conditions. *J Periodontol* **72**: 1790–800.

19. Meng HX (1999). Periodontal abscess. *Ann Periodontol* **4**: 79–83.

20. Bagg J, Sweeney MP, Harvey-Wood K, Wiggins A (1995). Possible role of *Staphylococcus aureus* in severe oral mucositis among elderly dehydrated patients. *Microb Ecol Health Dis* **8**: 51–6.

21. Gibson J, Wray D, Bagg J (2000). Oral staphylococcal mucositis: a new clinical entity in orofacial granulomatosis and Crohn's disease. *Oral Surg Oral Med Oral Pathol Oral Radiol Endod* **89**: 171–6.

22. Fattahi TT, Lyu PE, Van Sickels JE (2002). Management of acute suppurative parotitis. *J Oral Maxillofac Surg* **60**: 446–8.

Chapter 8

Viral infections

Jeremy Bagg

Introduction

A wide variety of viruses may cause oral infection.[1] However, the most important group of viruses is the herpes virus family. Hence, this chapter will concentrate on this group of viruses. Human immunodeficiency virus infection is discussed in detail in Chapter 16.

Viruses may cause isolated, or recurrent, infections. Moreover, viruses have been implicated in the pathogenesis of other oral pathologies, particularly of certain oral malignancies (Table 8.1).

Oral viral infections are a significant cause of morbidity amongst sick patients: the symptomatology includes specific problems (e.g. oral discomfort) as well as non-specific problems (e.g. malaise). It should be noted that oral infections may disseminate to cause systemic infections. Systemic viral infections are a significant cause of mortality amongst sick patients.

In most cases, the diagnosis of a viral infection rests on the clinical features. However, in immunosuppressed patients, the clinical features may be atypical. The methods used for detecting viruses include: (a) electron microscopy; (b) tissue culture; (c) antigen detection; (d) antibody detection; and (e) molecular methods (DNA hybridization, polymerase chain reaction).[1] Some methods are not applicable for diagnosing certain viral infections. Similarly, some methods are not applicable for providing urgent diagnoses (tissue culture). It is essential that the clinician liases with the microbiological laboratory about the most relevant method (and the specimens required to undertake that method).

Many viral infections do not require specific antiviral treatment. Nevertheless, patients should be prescribed appropriate symptomatic measures (antipyretics, analgesics). Herpes simplex virus/varicella zoster virus infections, particularly in immunosuppressed patients, usually require specific antiviral treatment (Table 8.2).[2] Generally, the dose of the drug needs increasing in immunosuppressed patients. Moreover, the route of administration of the drug may need changing in this group of patients, i.e. the drug may need to be given intravenously, rather than orally.

Table 8.1 Major viral infections involving the oral cavity[1]

Virus	Oral diseases/manifestations	Comments
Herpes simplex virus	Primary herpetic gingivostomatitis Herpes labialis (cold sore)	See text
Varicella zoster virus	Chicken pox – oral ulceration Shingles – oral ulceration	See text
Epstein–Barr virus (EBV)	Infectious mononucleosis – pharyngeal inflammation Oral hairy leukoplakia Nasopharyngeal carcinoma Burkitt's lymphoma	Oral hairy leukoplakia is discussed in detail in Chapter 16 EBV has been implicated in the pathogenesis of other malignancies, e.g. Hodgkin's disease
Measles virus	Measles – Koplik spots	Predominantly disease of childhood
Mumps virus	Mumps – salivary gland inflammation	Predominantly disease of childhood
Group A coxsackie viruses	Hand, foot and mouth disease Herpangina	Predominantly diseases of childhood
Human papilloma virus (HPV)	Verruca vulgaris (common wart) Condyloma acuminatum (venereal wart)	HPV has been implicated in the pathogenesis of certain malignancies, e.g. oral carcinoma
Human immunodeficiency virus (HIV)	Numerous oral manifestations	See Chapter 16

Table 8.2 Recommended treatment regimens for certain viral infections[2]

Viral infection	Recommended treatment regimens[2]	Comments
Secondary herpes simplex infection – herpes labialis	5% aciclovir cream – apply 4 hourly for 5–10 days 1% penciclovir cream – apply 2 hourly for 4 days	Available without prescription in UK Studies suggest this cream is more effective than aciclovir
Herpes simplex infection in immunocompromised patients	Aciclovir 400mg orally 5 times a day for 5 days or Aciclovir 5mg/kg iv 3 times a day for 5 days	Give IV in severe infections/severely immunosuppressed patients
Secondary varicella zoster infection – shingles	Aciclovir 800mg orally 5 times a day for 7 days Famciclovir 250mg orally 3 times a day for 7 days or Famciclovir 750mg orally once a day for 7 days Valaciclovir 1g orally 3 times a day for 7 days	Give IV in immunosuppressed patients Give larger dose in immunosuppressed patients These regimens may be more successful than aciclovir, because of improved drug concordance This regimen may be more successful than aciclovir, because of improved drug concordance

Herpes simplex virus (HSV) infections

All of the herpes viruses can establish latent infections. Latent herpes viruses may become reactivated in the immunocompetent, but reactivation is a particular problem among immunocompromised patients.

Primary herpes simplex infection – primary herpetic gingivostomatitis

Epidemiology

Primary herpetic gingivostomatitis is the most common viral infection of the mouth.

Aetiology

It is usually caused by HSV type I, though small number of cases are caused by HSV type II, which is the usual isolate from genital herpes.

Clinical features

Infection in early childhood often results in a subclinical infection, but in older children and adults the symptoms are more severe. Initially there is a fever, together with enlarged cervical lymph nodes and intra-oral pain. Vesicles then develop on the oral mucosa, particularly the gingiva, tongue and buccal mucosa. These vesicles are intra-epithelial and rupture quickly to form superficial ulcers with erythematous margins on greyish-yellow bases (Fig. 8.1). The mouth is painful, making eating and swallowing difficult. The lips may also be swollen and covered in a bloodstained crust.

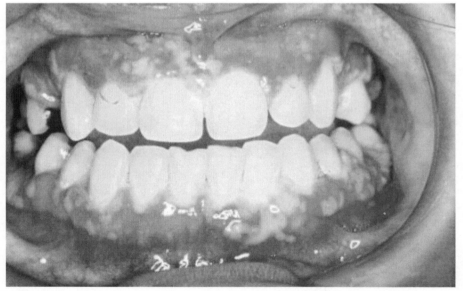

Fig. 8.1 Primary herpes simplex virus infection (primary herpetic gingivostomatitis). Reproduced with permission from MP Sweeney and J Bagg (1997), *Making Sense of the Mouth* Partnership in Oral Care, Glasgow. (See also Plate 20 at the centre of this book.)

Management

Bed rest, maintenance of fluid intake and provision of antipyretics are important elements of treatment. In the immunocompetent, the lesions are self-limiting and heal within 10 days without scarring. The prescribing of aciclovir at an early stage in the infection may shorten its course and reduce the severity of symptoms.[3]

Secondary (reactivation) herpes simplex infection – herpes labialis, other presentations

Epidemiology

About one-third of patients who have been infected with HSV develop secondary infections later in life, due to reactivation of virus lying latent in the trigeminal ganglion.

Aetiology

A number of factors have been associated with reactivation of HSV, including sun exposure and menstruation.

Clinical features

The most common lesion is herpes labialis, also known as a 'cold sore'. These lesions appear on the mucocutaneous junction of the lip, or on the skin adjacent to the nostril (Fig. 8.2). There is a premonitory burning sensation for 24 hours before the vesicles develop. The vesicles rupture, crust over and heal within 10–14 days.

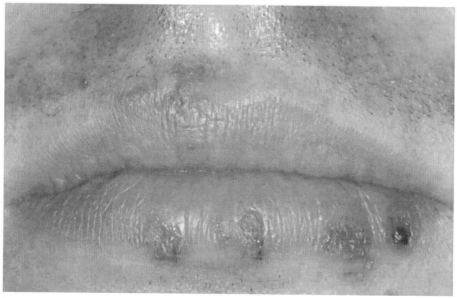

Fig. 8.2 Secondary herpes simplex virus infection in immunocompetent patient (herpes labialis). Courtesy of J Eveson. (See also Plate 21 at the centre of this book.)

Intra-oral reactivation lesions have been described, but are rare in the immuno-competent. They present as small clusters of lesions, typically involving the palatal mucosa.

Management

Treatment with topical application of 5 per cent aciclovir cream, starting during the premonitory burning sensation, may reduce the severity of the lesions (Table 8.2).[4] Recently, the efficacy of 1 per cent penciclovir cream has been demonstrated.[5] Indeed, this treatment appears currently to be the most effective topical agent for herpes labialis.[6]

Herpes simplex infection in immunocompromised patients

Clinical features

The clinical presentation is often atypical. The infection may present as either small crops of ulcers (Fig. 8.3), or as a more florid reaction (Fig. 8.4), both of which are very painful.

Management

Treatment should be commenced urgently with systemic aciclovir (Table 8.2).

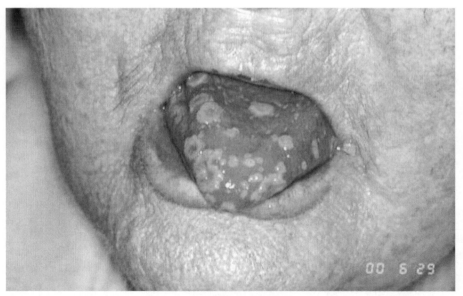

Fig. 8.3 Secondary herpes simplex virus infection in immunocompromised patient. Courtesy of MP Sweeney. (See also Plate 22 at the centre of this book.)

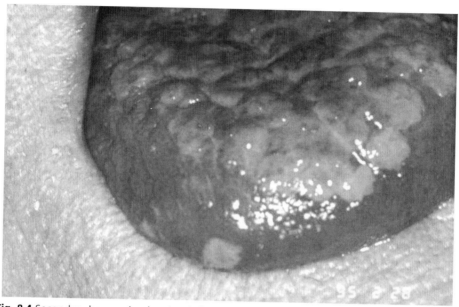

Fig. 8.4 Secondary herpes simplex virus infection in immunocompromised patient. Reproduced with permission from MP Sweeney and J Bagg (1997), *Making Sense of the Mouth* Partnership in Oral Care, Glasgow. (See also Plate 23 at the centre of this book.)

Varicella zoster virus infections

Primary varicella zoster infection – chicken pox

Clinical features

Before development of the skin rash, oral lesions may be detectable, especially on the hard palate, pillars of the fauces, and uvula. The oral lesions are small ulcers, 2–4mm in diameter, surrounded by an erythematous halo.

Secondary (reactivation) varicella zoster infection – shingles

Epidemiology

Shingles is more common in older individuals.

Aetiology

It results from reactivation of varicella zoster virus lying latent in sensory ganglia. Cellular immune dysfunction can trigger shingles, for example HIV infection, Hodgkin's disease, non-Hodgkin's lymphoma, and bone marrow or solid organ transplants.

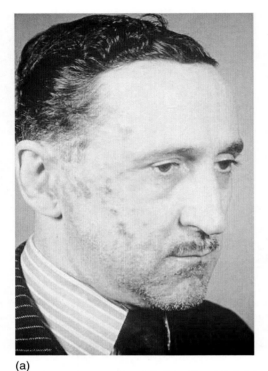

(a)

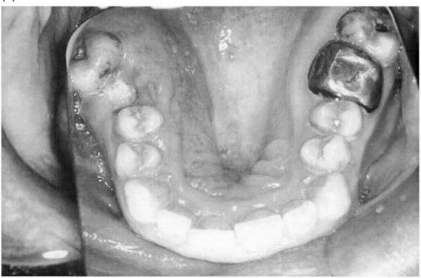

(b)

Fig. 8.5 (a) Secondary varicella zoster (facial component). **(b)** Secondary varicella zoster (oral component). Reproduced with permission from MP Sweeney and J Bagg (1997), *Making Sense of the Mouth*, Partnership in Oral Care, Glasgow. (See also Plates 24(a) and (b) at the centre of this book.)

Clinical features

Local severe pain and paraesthesia commonly precede the appearance of the skin eruption by several days. The skin lesions present as a localized eruption involving an area of skin supplied by one or more sensory ganglia (dermatome). Groups of vesicles are present on an erythematous base, and the distribution is almost invariably unilateral. The vesicles dry within a few days to form scabs, which separate and heal without scarring. The trigeminal nerve is involved in about 15 per cent of cases. If the maxillary or mandibular divisions are affected, then the lesions of shingles may affect both skin and oral mucosa (Figs 8.5(a) and (b)). Subsequently a proportion of patients, particularly the elderly, may suffer from an intractable form of pain known as post-herpetic neuralgia.

Management

High dose aciclovir, famciclovir, or valaciclovir are all acceptable antiviral drugs for treatment, and should be prescribed as soon as possible (Table 8.2).[7] Corticosteroids, in conjunction with antiviral treatment, have been shown to have a beneficial effect.[8] Analgesics are also necessary for achieving pain control.

Other herpes virus infections

Epstein–Barr virus

Epstein–Barr virus is associated with a variety of oral problems, including infectious mononucleosis, oral hairy leukoplakia (see Chapter 16, Fig. 16.3), nasopharyngeal carcinoma, and Burkitt's lymphoma.[9] It should be noted that although oral hairy leukoplakia is a common manifestation of HIV infection/AIDS, it has been reported in HIV-negative immunosuppressed patients,[10] and also in HIV-negative immunocompetent patients.[11]

Cytomegalovirus

Cytomegalovirus has been shown to be the cause of oral ulceration in HIV-positive patients,[12] and also in HIV-negative immunosuppressed patients.[13]

Human herpes virus 8

Human herpes virus 8 is associated with Kaposi's sarcoma (see Chapter 16, Fig. 16.6).[14]

References

1. Bagg J, MacFarlane TW, Poxton IR, Miller CH, Smith AJ (1999). *Essentials of Microbiology for Dental Students*. Oxford: Oxford University Press.
2. Anonymous (2003). *British National Formulary* 46 (September 2003). London: British Medical Association and the Royal Pharmaceutical Society of Great Britain.
3. Amir J (2001). Clinical aspects and antiviral therapy in primary herpetic gingivostomatitis. *Paediatr Drugs* **3**: 593–7.

4. Spruance SL, Nett R, Marbury T, Wolff R, Johnson J, Spaulding T (2002). Acyclovir cream for treatment of herpes simplex labialis: results of two randomized, double-blind, vehicle-controlled, multicenter clinical trials. *Antimicrob Agents Chemother* **46**: 2238–43.

5. Raborn GW, Martel AY, Lassonde M, Lewis MA, Boon R, Spruance SL (2002). Worldwide Topical Penciclovir Collaborative Study Group. Effective treatment of herpes simplex labialis with penciclovir cream: combined results of two trials. *J Am Dent Assoc* **133**: 303–9.

6. Vander Straten M, Carrasco D, Lee P, Tyring SK (2001). A review of antiviral therapy for herpes labialis. *Arch Dermatol* **137**: 1232–5.

7. Schmader K (2001). Herpes zoster in older adults. *Clin Infect Dis* **32**: 1481–6.

8. Johnson RW, Dworkin RH (2003). Treatment of herpes zoster and postherpetic neuralgia. *BMJ* **326**: 748–50.

9. Cruchley AT, Williams DM, Niedobitek G, Young LS (1997). Epstein–Barr virus: biology and disease. *Oral Dis* **3** Suppl 1: S156–63.

10. Seymour RA, Thomason JM, Nolan A (1997). Oral lesions in organ transplant patients. *J Oral Pathol Med* **26**: 297–304.

11. Felix DH, Watret K, Wray D, Southam JC (1992). Hairy leukoplakia in an HIV-negative, nonimmunosuppressed patient. *Oral Surg Oral Med Oral Pathol* **74**: 563–6.

12. Syrjanen S, Leimola-Virtanen R, Schmidt-Westhausen A, Reichart PA (1999). Oral ulcers in AIDS patients frequently associated with cytomegalovirus (CMV) and Epstein–Barr virus (EBV) infections. *J Oral Pathol Med* **28**: 204–9.

13. Epstein J, Scully C (1993). Cytomegalovirus: a virus of increasing relevance to oral medicine and pathology. *J Oral Pathol Med* **22**: 348–53.

14. Geraminejad P, Memar O, Aronson I, Rady PL, Hengge U, Tyring SK (2002). Kaposi's sarcoma and other manifestations of human herpesvirus 8. *J Am Acad Dermatol* **47**: 641–55.

Useful websites

International Herpes Management Forum
http://www.ihmf.org

Chapter 9

Salivary gland dysfunction

Andrew Davies

Anatomy and physiology

The salivary glands are divided into two main groups:

- Major salivary glands.

There are six major salivary glands: two parotid glands, two submandibular glands and two sublingual glands (Fig. 9.1).

- Minor salivary glands.

There are hundreds of minor salivary glands, situated in the tongue, the palate, the buccal mucosa and the labial mucosa.

The secretion of saliva is predominantly controlled by the parasympathetic nervous system. Thus, stimulation of the parasympathetic nervous system leads to an increase in the secretion of saliva, whilst inhibition of the parasympathetic nervous system leads to a decrease in the secretion of saliva. The sympathetic nervous system can also affect saliva secretion. The sympathetic nervous system is mainly concerned with the composition of saliva secreted, rather than with the volume of saliva secreted.

The 'unstimulated' (resting) salivary flow rate is affected by a number of factors, including:[1]

- Degree of hydration – subjects who are dehydrated have a decreased salivary flow rate. Indeed, if the total body water content falls by 8 per cent, then the salivary flow rate falls to zero.[2]

- Body posture – salivary flow rate is highest when standing, is intermediate when sitting, and is lowest when lying down.

- Exposure to light – salivary flow rate decreases by 30–40 per cent when subjects are placed in the dark.[2]

- Circadian rhythms – salivary flow rate is highest in the late afternoon, and is lowest in the night.

Eating is the predominant cause of salivary gland stimulation, i.e. increased secretion of saliva. Food stimulates gustatory, touch, and pressure receptors in the mouth, which feedback to the parasympathetic nervous system. Furthermore, mastication of the food stimulates pressure and proprioception receptors in the surrounding tissues

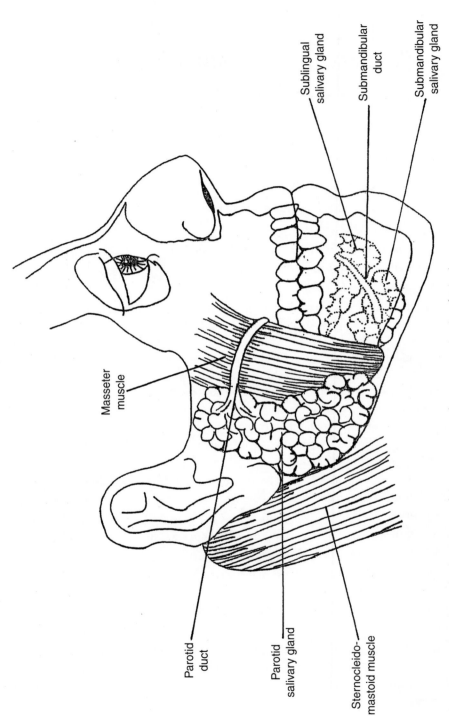

Fig. 9.1 The major salivary glands. Courtesy of the Department of Anatomy, University of Bristol.

(periodontal ligament, muscles of mastication, temporomandibular joint), which also feed back to the parasympathetic nervous system. Other relevant stimuli include the smell of food (via olfactory receptors in the nose), and the sight of food (via higher centres in the brain).

The 'stimulated' salivary flow rate is also affected by a number of factors, including:

◆ Consistency of food – food with a firm consistency causes a greater increase in salivary flow than food with a soft consistency.

◆ Taste of food – food with strong flavours causes a greater increase in salivary flow than food with bland flavours.

◆ Other characteristics of food, e.g. pH.

It has been calculated that the average person produces 500–600 ml of saliva per day.[2] At rest, the submandibular glands contribute ~ 65 per cent, the parotid glands ~ 20 per cent, the sublingual glands ~ 7–8 per cent, and the minor salivary glands ~ 7–8 per cent of the salivary gland output.[2] However, during periods of stimulation, the parotid gland contribution increases to ~ 50 per cent of the total. The individual salivary glands produce secretions with a slightly different protein composition. For example, the minor salivary glands produce secretions rich in mucin. Indeed, the minor salivary glands contribute ~ 70 per cent of the total mucin content of whole saliva.[3]

Ninety-nine percent of saliva is water.[4] The remaining one percent consists of a variety of electrolytes, small organic molecules and large organic molecules (Table 9.1). The diverse constituents of saliva reflect the diverse functions of saliva (Table 9.2).[4] The composition of saliva is affected by a number of factors, including the salivary flow rate, and the composition of plasma.[2] It should be noted that there are a number of other components of saliva, including gingival crevicular fluid, epithelial cells, serum, blood cells, various organisms, and food debris.[4]

Table 9.1 Composition of saliva

Class of molecule	Specific molecules
Electrolytes	Ammonia, bicarbonate, calcium, chloride, fluoride, iodide, magnesium, phosphates, potassium, sodium, sulphates, thiocyanate
Small organic molecules	Creatinine, glucose, nitrogen, sialic acid, urea, uric acid
Large organic molecules	Albumin, amylase, ß-glucuronidase, carbohydrases, cystatins, epidermal growth factor, esterases, fibronectin, gustin, histatins, immunoglobulin A, immunoglobulin G, immunoglobulin M, kallikrein, lactic dehydrogenase, lactoferrin, lipase, lipids, lysozyme, mucins, nerve growth factor, parotid aggregins, peptidases, phosphatases, proline-rich proteins, ribonucleases, salivary peroxidases, tyrosine-rich proteins, vitamin-binding proteins

Table 9.2 Functions of saliva

Function	Components responsible for function
Lubrication	Water, mucins, proline-rich proteins
Mucosal integrity	Water, electrolytes, mucins
Antimicrobial	Cystatins, histatins, Ig A, lactoferrin, lactoperoxidase, lysozyme, mucins, proline-rich proteins
Lavage/cleansing	Water
Buffering	Bicarbonate, phosphates
Remineralization (of teeth)	Calcium, phosphates, proline-rich proteins, tyrosine-rich proteins
Food preparation	Water, mucins
Digestion	Water, amylase, lipase, mucins, peptidases, ribonucleases
Taste	Water, gustin
Speech	Water, mucins

Definitions

Xerostomia has been defined as 'the subjective sensation of dryness of the mouth',[5] whilst salivary gland hypofunction has been defined as 'any objectively demonstrable reduction in either whole and/or individual gland flow rates'.[6] Xerostomia is usually the result of a decrease in the volume of saliva secreted. Indeed, normal subjects usually complain of a dry mouth when their unstimulated whole salivary flow rate falls by 50 per cent.[1] However, xerostomia may also result from a change in the composition of the saliva secreted.[4] Salivary gland dysfunction (SGD) has been used as an umbrella term to describe patients with xerostomia and/or salivary gland hypofunction (Fig. 9.2).

Epidemiology

The prevalence of xerostomia in the general population has been reported to be between 22–26 per cent.[8,9] Xerostomia is more common in patients with chronic illness[10] and the prevalence of xerostomia in the palliative care population has been reported to be between 29–77 per cent.[11,12] However, studies have generally reported that the prevalence of xerostomia is >50 per cent in this group of patients.[13,14] Indeed, studies have generally reported that xerostomia is one of the five most common symptoms in this group of patients.[13,15] The prevalence of salivary gland hypofunction in the palliative care population has been reported to be between 82–83 per cent.[16,17]

Aetiology

The most common cause for SGD in the general population is drug treatment.[18] There are a large number of drugs that can produce SGD.[19] Indeed, 63 per cent of

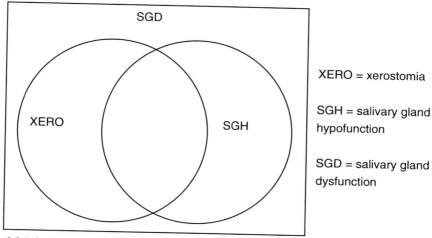

Fig. 9.2 Relationship between xerostomia, salivary gland hypofunction and salivary gland dysfunction.

the 200 most frequently prescribed drugs in the US during 1992 were drugs that can produce this complication.[20] Drugs cause SGD via a number of different mechanisms.[21] The direct effects include interference with the nervous supply of the salivary glands (e.g. anticholinergic effect of antidepressants), or with the productive capacity of salivary glands (e.g. dehydrating effect of diuretics). The indirect effects include interference with the normal stimuli to the secretion of saliva, e.g. impairment of the sensation of taste. The most common cause of SGD in the palliative care population is also drug treatment.[15,17]

There are numerous other causes of SGD in the general population.[4] Interestingly, the most common cause in patients attending specialist oral medicine clinics is Sjögren's syndrome.[22] Sjögren's syndrome is an autoimmune condition, which may occur in isolation (primary Sjögren's syndrome), or in conjunction with a connective disease disorder (secondary Sjögren's syndrome).[23] It is characterized by the presence of SGD, and lacrimal gland dysfunction (dry eyes). There are also numerous other causes of SGD in the palliative care population (Fig. 9.3).

SGD is a predictable side-effect of radiotherapy to the head and neck region.[24] It develops soon after the initiation of treatment, progresses during treatment (and for some time after treatment), and is essentially permanent. SGD can also be a side-effect of radioiodine therapy.[25]

Clinical features

SGD is associated with a variety of different oral problems. Moreover, SGD may result in a more generalised deterioration in the patient's physical and psychological condition. The oral problems encountered in SGD reflect the various functions of saliva (Table 9.2).

Disease of/damage to salivary glands
- ■ Related to cancer – tumour infiltration, paraneoplastic syndrome
- ■ Related to cancer treatment – surgery, radiotherapy, chemotherapy, graft versus host disease
- ■ Unrelated to cancer – e.g. Sjögren's syndrome

Damage to/interference with autonomic nerve supply of salivary glands
- ■ Related to cancer – tumour infiltration
- ■ Related to cancer treatment – surgery, radiotherapy
- ■ Unrelated to cancer – e.g. dementia

Interference with productive capacity of salivary glands
- ■ Dehydration
- ■ Malnutrition

Miscellaneous
- ■ Drug treatment
- ■ Decreased oral intake
- ■ Decreased mastication
- ■ Anxiety
- ■ Depression

Fig. 9.3 Aetiology of salivary gland dysfunction in patients with advanced cancer.

The symptoms associated with SGD include:[8,26]

- ◆ Xerostomia. The xerostomia can be continuous, or intermittent; it can lead to insomnia.
- ◆ Oral discomfort. The oral discomfort can be generalized, or localized; it can be non-specific, 'burning', or 'tingling' in nature; it can lead to difficulty wearing dental prostheses ('dentures').
- ◆ Lip discomfort.
- ◆ Impairment of sensation of taste (dysgeusia).
- ◆ Difficulty chewing (dysmasesia).
- ◆ Difficulty swallowing (dysphagia).
- ◆ Difficulty speaking (dysphonia).

The signs associated with SGD include:[6,8]

- ◆ Dryness of the mucous membranes.
- ◆ Dryness of the lips.
- ◆ No 'pool' of saliva in the floor of the mouth.

- Fissuring of the tongue.
- Dental caries.

SGD is associated with the development of new lesions, rapidly progressive lesions, and lesions in unusual sites (e.g. the lower anterior teeth).[5]

- Oral candidosis.
- Other oral infections.

Patients with SGD can have some, or all of the above clinical features. Indeed, patients can be asymptomatic, but have clinical signs of SGD. Similarly, patients can be symptomatic, but have no clinical signs of SGD.

The psychosocial effects of SGD include shame, increased feelings of being a patient rather than a person, and a tendency to avoid social contact.[27] These issues are highlighted by a quote from one of the patients in the Rydholm and Strang study.[27]:

> Earlier before this I used to participate in choir singing, nowadays I can't sing at all because my voice is so weak, my vocal cords are so dry and I am afraid to 'lose my head', so I won't participate at all, I avoid all these things and prefer staying at home. I feel sorry and depressed.

Investigations

The diagnosis of SGD can usually be made on clinical criteria, i.e. history and examination.[6] Sialometry (measurement of salivary flow rates) is not usually indicated in palliative care practice. Similarly, other investigations are not usually indicated in palliative care practice e.g. sialochemistry (biochemical analysis of saliva), sialography (X-ray imaging of salivary glands) and scintigraphy (radioisotope imaging of salivary glands).[4] Investigations for diagnosing Sjögren's syndrome include measurement of certain serum autoantibodies and histological examination of a labial biopsy.[23]

Techniques have been developed to measure unstimulated salivary flow rates (usual flow rates), stimulated salivary flow rates (postprandial flow rates), salivary flow from all of the glands ('whole' salivary flow rates), and salivary flow from individual glands. The most clinically relevant salivary flow rates are the unstimulated whole salivary flow rate (UWSFR), and the stimulated whole salivary flow rate (SWSFR). The presence of xerostomia is more closely related to the UWSFR than to the SWSFR.[15,28]

Management

The management of SGD involves:

- Treatment of the cause
- Symptomatic treatment
- Treatment of the complications.

Generally, it is not possible to treat the cause of the SGD. As stated above, the most common cause of SGD is drug treatment. In theory, it is possible to discontinue, or substitute, the relevant drugs. However, in practice, it is usually very difficult to discontinue, or substitute, all of the relevant drugs. Thus, Davies *et al.* reported that patients were taking a median of 4 (range of 0–9) such drugs, and that many of these drugs were necessary for symptom control.[15,17] Moreover, SGD is usually a drug class side-effect, rather than an individual drug side-effect.[19]

The symptomatic treatment of SGD involves the use of either saliva substitutes, or saliva stimulants.[29] Most studies have been performed in patients with non-malignant disease, and a good performance status. However, there have been some studies performed in typical palliative care patients (i.e. patients with malignant disease, and a poor performance status). The results of relevant randomized controlled trials involving saliva substitutes are shown in Table 9.3,[30–32] whilst the results of relevant randomized controlled trials involving saliva stimulants are shown in Table 9.4.[31,32]

Saliva substitutes

Water

Patients commonly use water. However, in clinical trials, patients have reported that water was less effective than other saliva substitutes (artificial saliva).[33,34] Moreover, in one study, the mean duration of subjective improvement with water was only 12 min (range 4–29 min).[35]

In spite of the above, many patients persevere with water. The use of water may be associated with polyuria (and nocturia).

Artificial saliva

Health care professionals commonly prescribe 'artificial saliva'. Several different types of artificial saliva have been developed: these products differ in the lubricant used (mucin, cellulose, other), the formulations available (spray, gel, other) and the additives used (fluoride, antimicrobial factors, other).

In clinical trials, patients have reported that mucin-based artificial saliva was more effective, and better tolerated, than cellulose-based artificial saliva.[36,37] In other clinical trials, patients have reported that some other types of artificial saliva (polyacrylic acid-based; xanthan gum-based) were as effective as the mucin-based artificial saliva.[38] Interestingly, patients have also reported that gel-based artificial saliva was more effective than spray-based artificial saliva.[39] The results of studies involving palliative care patients are shown in Table 9.3. It should be noted that the availability of the different saliva substitutes varies from country to country.

The 'ideal' artificial saliva should have a neutral pH (to prevent demineralisation of the teeth), and contain fluoride (to enhance remineralization of the teeth). Some commercial artificial saliva has an acidic pH, and, therefore, should not be prescribed for dentate patients.[7] The addition of flavourings may enhance the efficacy of

Table 9.3 Randomized controlled trials (RCT) of saliva substitutes in the palliative care setting

Study	Treatment	Effectiveness of treatment	Side-effects of treatment	Other comments
Sweeney et al. 1997[30]	Mucin-based artificial saliva prn	Improvement in xerostomia in 60% of patients	Side-effects: none reported	RCT: mucin-based artificial saliva vs 'placebo' spray 93% of patients wanted to continue with artificial saliva
Davies et al. 1998[31]	Mucin-based artificial saliva qds	Improvement in xerostomia in 73% of patients	Side-effects: 31% of patients; nausea, diarrhoea, irritation of mouth	RCT: mucin-based artificial saliva vs pilocarpine 64% of patients wanted to continue with artificial saliva
Davies 2000[32]	Mucin-based artificial saliva qds	Improvement in xerostomia in 89% of patients	Side-effects: 19% of patients; nausea, unpleasant taste, irritation of mouth	RCT: mucin-based artificial saliva vs chewing gum 74% of patients wanted to continue with artificial saliva

Table 9.4 Randomized controlled trials of saliva stimulants in the palliative care setting

Study	Treatment	Effectiveness of treatment	Side-effects of treatment	Other comments
Davies et al. 1998[31]	Pilocarpine 5mg tds	Improvement in xerostomia in 90% of patients	Side-effects: 84% of patients; sweating, dizziness, lacrimation	RCT: mucin-based artificial saliva vs pilocarpine. 76% of patients wanted to continue with pilocarpine. Pilocarpine more effective than mucin-based artificial saliva.
Davies 2000[32]	Chewing gum 1–2 pieces qds	Improvement in xerostomia in 90% of patients	Side-effects: 22% of patients; irritation of mouth, nausea, unpleasant taste	RCT: mucin-based artificial saliva vs chewing gum. 86% of patients wanted to continue with chewing gum. Chewing gum as effective as mucin-based artificial saliva. (Patients preferred chewing gum)

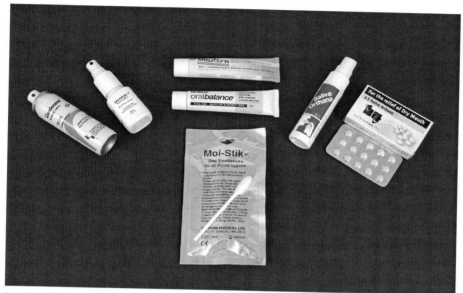

Fig. 9.4 Saliva substitutes available in United Kingdom.

the product by actually stimulating the secretion of saliva. Similarly, the addition of antibacterial agents (particularly lactoperoxidase) may enhance the efficacy of the product by inhibiting the growth of pathogens.[40]

In spite of the above, many patients do not persevere with artificial saliva.[41] The use of artificial saliva may be associated with local irritation, and various other side-effects (Table 9.3).

Other agents

Other agents that have been used as saliva substitutes include milk, butter, vegetable oil and margarine.[42–44]

Glycerine, often used in combination with lemon, has been recommended as a saliva substitute. However, this agent actually causes dryness of the mouth.[45]

Saliva stimulants

Chewing gum

Chewing gum increases salivary flow mainly through stimulation of chemoreceptors (taste effect; ~85 per cent of action), and partly through stimulation of mechanoreceptors (chewing effect; ~15 per cent of action).[46]

Chewing gum has been shown to be effective in the management of xerostomia in various groups of patients,[29] including patients with advanced cancer (Table 9.4).[32]

Moreover, chewing gum has been shown to be more effective than artificial saliva, and other saliva stimulants (organic acids).[47–48] Chewing gum is an acceptable form of treatment to most patients, including to most elderly patients.[32,49] Patients with SGD should use 'sugar-free' chewing gum, whilst patients with dental prostheses should use 'low-tack' (less sticky) chewing gum.

Chewing gum is generally well tolerated. Side-effects may be related to: (a) chewing, e.g. jaw discomfort, headache; (b) ingestion, e.g. respiratory tract obstruction, gastrointestinal obstruction; (c) non-allergic reactions to additives, e.g. oral discomfort, flatulence; (d) allergic reactions to additives, e.g. stomatitis, perioral dermatitis.[32]

Organic acids

Various organic acids have been used as saliva stimulants, including ascorbic acid (vitamin C), citric acid (acid from citrus fruits), and malic acid (acid from apples and pears). The organic acids increase salivary flow through stimulation of chemoreceptors.

Ascorbic acid has been found to be somewhat ineffective: in the Bjornstrom study[47] only 33 per cent of the patients rated ascorbic acid as either 'good' or 'very good', and only 23 per cent of patients wanted to continue with it after the study. Similarly, citric acid has been shown to be less useful than artificial saliva and chewing gum.[48] Malic acid has been found to be somewhat more effective: in the Bjornstrom study[47] 51 per cent of the patients rated malic acid as either 'good' or 'very good', and 44 per cent of patients wanted to continue with it after the study.

The use of organic acids is associated with oral discomfort[48] and demineralization of the teeth.[50] Thus, organic acids should not be used in patients with mucositis, or patients with their own teeth.

Parasympathomimetic drugs

These drugs, which are either choline esters, or cholinesterase inhibitors, act via the parasympathetic nervous supply to the salivary glands.

Pilocarpine is a choline ester, which primarily acts on muscarinic receptors. However, pilocarpine also acts on beta-adrenergic receptors.[51] Pilocarpine has been shown to be effective in the management of SGD secondary to various causes, including drug treatment,[31] salivary gland disease[52] and (particularly) radiotherapy.[53,54] Moreover, pilocarpine has been shown to be more effective than artificial saliva in the management of SGD secondary to drug treatment[31] and radiotherapy.[55]

The response to pilocarpine appears to depend to a certain extent on the aetiology of the SGD. Thus, most patients with SGD secondary to drugs or salivary gland disease report an improvement in symptoms,[31,52] whilst only ~ 50 per cent of patients with SGD secondary to radiotherapy report an improvement in symptoms.[53,54] In most patients the response to treatment is immediate.[52] However, in patients with radiation-induced SGD the response to treatment may not occur for many (up to 12) weeks.[53,54]

The side-effects of pilocarpine are usually the result of generalized parasympathetic stimulation. The most common side-effects are sweating, urinary frequency, headache, vasodilation, nausea, dizziness, dyspepsia, rhinorrhoea and fatigue.[56] The incidence of side-effects is dose dependent. For example, the incidence of sweating is 29 per cent at a dose of 5mg three times a day, and 68 per cent at a dose of 10mg three times a day.[56]

Other parasympathomimetic drugs have been used in the management of salivary gland dysfunction, including:

1. Choline esters – bethanechol,[57] cevimeline.[58]
2. Cholinesterase inhibitors – distigmine,[29] pyridostigmine.[29]

Acupuncture

The precise mechanism of action of acupuncture has not been elucidated. However, it is known to increase the secretion of certain neuropeptides, and to increase the flow of blood within the oral cavity.[59]

Acupuncture has been reported to be effective in the management of SGD secondary to drug treatment,[59] radiotherapy[60] and Sjögren's syndrome.[61] However, most of the evidence is derived from uncontrolled studies, or from studies comparing acupuncture with 'placebo' acupuncture. It should be noted that the study by Rydholm and Strang was conducted in the palliative care setting.[59]

Investigators have used diverse acupuncture points (number/type of points), and diverse treatment schedules (number/duration of treatment). Indeed, there is no

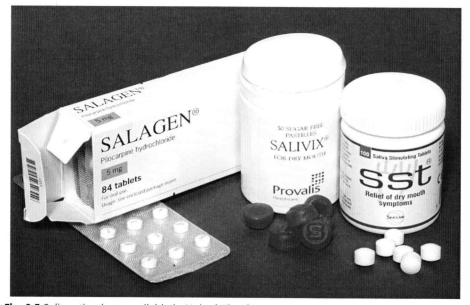

Fig. 9.5 Saliva stimulants available in United Kingdom.

standard treatment regimen. The effect of acupuncture may be delayed[59] but may also be long-lasting (continue after the end of treatment).[60,61] The effect of acupuncture may be maintained by intermittent retreatment.[60]

Acupuncture is generally well tolerated. Nevertheless, it can lead to local haemorrhage, and also to local/systemic infection. Thus, acupuncture should be used with caution in patients with bleeding diatheses, and patients that are immunocompromised. Patients have reported feeling tired after treatment.[61]

Interestingly, some patients report that their other symptoms improve after treatment (pain, insomnia).[61] Moreover, some patients report that they feel non-specifically 'better' after treatment.[61]

Other agents

A number of other pharmacological means have been used, including anetho-letrithione,[62] nicotinamide (B group vitamin)[47] and yohimbine (alpha 2 adrenore-ceptor antagonist).[63] Similarly, a number of other non-pharmacological means have been used, including 'sugar-free' sweets[46] and a device called an 'electrostimulator'.[64]

Complementary therapies are another therapeutic option, particularly homeopathy, and Chinese medicine.[65]

The choice of symptomatic treatment will depend on a number of factors, including the aetiology of the xerostomia, the patient's general condition and prognosis, the presence or absence of teeth and, most importantly, the patient's preference.

There are good theoretical reasons for prescribing saliva stimulants rather than saliva substitutes. The saliva stimulants cause an increase in secretion of normal saliva, and so will ameliorate both xerostomia and the other complications of SGD.[53–55] In contrast, the saliva substitutes will generally only ameliorate xerostomia.[55] Furthermore, in the studies that have compared salivary stimulants with saliva substitutes, patients have generally preferred the salivary stimulants.[47] Nevertheless, some patients do not respond to saliva stimulants, e.g. some patients with radiation-induced SGD.

The management of SGD also involves general oral hygiene measures (see Chapter 3), the use of fluoride supplements, and general dental care measures (dental cleaning, dental restoration).[7]

References

1. Dawes C (1987). Physiological factors affecting salivary flow rate, oral sugar clearance, and the sensation of dry mouth in man. *J Dent Res* **66**: 648–53.
2. Dawes C (1996). Factors influencing salivary flow rate and composition. In WM Edgar and DM O'Mullane (ed.) *Saliva and Oral Health*, 2nd edn, pp. 27–41. London: British Dental Association.
3. Tabak LA, Levine MJ, Mandel ID, Ellison SA (1982). Role of salivary mucins in the protection of the oral cavity. *J Oral Pathol* **11**: 1–17.
4. Anonymous (1992). Saliva: its role in health and disease. FDI Working Group 10 of the Commission on Oral Health, Research and Epidemiology (CORE). *Int Dent J* **42** (Suppl 2): 291–304.

5. Sreebny LM (1996). Xerostomia: diagnosis, management and clinical complications. In WM Edgar and DM O'Mullane (ed.) *Saliva and Oral Health*, 2nd edn, pp. 43–66. London: British Dental Association.

6. Navazesh M, Christensen C, Brightman V (1992). Clinical criteria for the diagnosis of salivary gland hypofunction. *J Dent Res* **71**: 1363–9.

7. Pankhurst CL, Smith EC, Rogers JO, Dunne SM, Jackson SHD, Proctor G (1996). Diagnosis and management of the dry mouth: part 1. *Dent Update* **23**: 56–62.

8. Billings RJ, Proskin HM, Moss ME (1996). Xerostomia and associated factors in a community-dwelling adult population. *Community Dent Oral Epidemiol* **24**: 312–16.

9. Nederfors T, Isaksson R, Mornstad H, Dahlof C (1997). Prevalence of perceived symptoms of dry mouth in an adult Swedish population – relation to age, sex and pharmacotherapy. *Community Dent Oral Epidemiol* **25**: 211–16.

10. Johnson G, Barenthin I, Westphal P (1984). Mouthdryness among patients in longterm hospitals. *Gerodontol* **3**: 197–203.

11. Maltoni M, Pirovano M, Scarpi E, Marinari M, Indelli M, Arnoldi E et al. (1995). Prediction of survival of patients terminally ill with cancer. *Cancer* **75**: 2613–22.

12. Jobbins J, Bagg J, Finlay IG, Addy M, Newcombe RG (1992). Oral and dental disease in terminally ill cancer patients. *BMJ* **304**: 1612.

13. Reuben DB, Mor V, Hiris J (1988). Clinical symptoms and length of survival in patients with terminal cancer. *Arch Intern Med* **148**: 1586–91.

14. Conill C, Verger E, Henriquez I, Saiz N, Espier M, Lugo F et al. (1997). Symptom prevalence in the last week of life. *J Pain Symptom Manage* **14**: 328–31.

15. Davies AN, Broadley K, Beighton D (2001). Xerostomia in patients with advanced cancer. *J Pain Symptom Manage* **22**: 820–5.

16. Chaushu G, Bercovici M, Dori S, Waller A, Taicher S, Kronenberg J et al. (2000). Salivary flow and its relation with oral symptoms in terminally ill patients. *Cancer* **88**: 984–7.

17. Davies AN, Broadley K, Beighton D (2002). Salivary gland hypofunction in patients with advanced cancer. *Oral Oncol* **38**: 680–5.

18. Sreebny LM, Valdini A, Yu A (1989). Xerostomia. Part II: Relationship to nonoral symptoms, drugs, and diseases. *Oral Surg Oral Med Oral Pathol* **68**: 419–27.

19. Sreebny LM, Schwartz SS (1997). A reference guide to drugs and dry mouth-2nd edn. *Gerodontology* **14**: 33–47.

20. Smith RG, Burtner AP (1994). Oral side-effects of the most frequently prescribed drugs. *Spec Care Dentist* **14**: 96–102.

21. Schubert MM, Izutsu KT (1987). Iatrogenic causes of salivary gland dysfunction. *J Dent Res* **66** (Spec Iss): 680–8.

22. Field EA, Longman LP, Bucknall R, Kaye SB, Higham SM, Edgar WM (1997). The establishment of a xerostomia clinic: a prospective study. *Br J Oral Maxillofac Surg* **35**: 96–103.

23. Vitali C, Bombardieri S, Jonsson R, Moutsopoulos HM, Alexander EL, Carsons SE et al. (2002). Classification criteria for Sjögren's syndrome: a revised version of the European criteria proposed by the American – European Consensus Group. *Ann Rheum Dis* **61**: 554–8.

24. Guchelaar HJ, Vermes A, Meerwaldt JH (1997). Radiation-induced xerostomia: pathophysiology, clinical course and supportive treatment. *Support Care Cancer* **5**: 281–8.

25. Solans R, Bosch JA, Galofre P, Porta F, Rosello J, Selva-O'Callagan A, et al. (2001). Salivary and lacrimal gland dysfunction (sicca syndrome) after radioiodine therapy. *J Nucl Med* **42**: 738–43.

26. Sreebny LM, Valdini A (1988). Xerostomia. Part I: Relationship to other oral symptoms and salivary gland hypofunction. *Oral Surg Oral Med Oral Pathol* **66**: 451–8.

27. Rydholm M, Strang P (2002). Physical and psychosocial impact of xerostomia in palliative cancer care: a qualitative interview study. *Int J Palliat Nurs* **8**: 318–23.

28. Wang SL, Zhao ZT, Li J, Zhu XZ, Dong H, Zhang YG (1998). Investigation of the clinical value of total saliva flow rates. *Arch Oral Biol* **43**: 39–43.

29. Davies AN (1997). The management of xerostomia: a review. *Eur J Cancer Care* **6**: 209–14.

30. Sweeney MP, Bagg J, Baxter WP, Aitchison TC (1997). Clinical trial of a mucin-containing oral spray for treatment of xerostomia in hospice patients. *Palliat Med* **11**: 225–32.

31. Davies AN, Daniels C, Pugh R, Sharma K (1998). A comparison of artificial saliva and pilocarpine in the management of xerostomia in patients with advanced cancer. *Palliat Med* **12**: 105–11.

32. Davies AN (2000). A comparison of artificial saliva and chewing gum in the management of xerostomia in patients with advanced cancer. *Palliat Med* **14**: 197–203.

33. Duxbury AJ, Thakker NS, Wastell DG (1989). A double-blind cross-over trial of a mucin-containing artificial saliva. *Br Dent J* **166**: 115–20.

34. Wiesenfeld D, Stewart AM, Mason DK (1983). A critical assessment of oral lubricants in patients with xerostomia. *Br Dent J* **155**: 155–7.

35. Olsson H, Axell T (1991). Objective and subjective efficacy of saliva substitutes containing mucin and carboxymethylcellulose. *Scand J Dent Res* **99**: 316–19.

36. Vissink A, 's-Gravenmade EJ, Panders AK, Vermey A, Petersen JK, Visch LL, et al. (1983). A clinical comparison between commercially available mucin- and CMC-containing saliva substitutes. *Int J Oral Surg* **12**: 232–8.

37. Visch LL, 's-Gravenmade EJ, Schaub RMH, Van Putten WLJ, Vissink A (1986). A double-blind crossover trial of CMC- and mucin-containing saliva substitutes. *Int J Oral Maxillofac Surg* **15**: 395–400.

38. Van der Reijden WA, van der Kwaak H, Vissink A, Veerman ECI, Nieuw Amerongen AV (1996). Treatment of xerostomia with polymer-based saliva substitutes in patients with Sjögren's syndrome. *Arthritis Rheum* **39**: 57–63.

39. Furumoto EK, Barker GJ, Carter-Hanson C, Barker BF (1998). Subjective and clinical evaluation of oral lubricants in xerostomic patients. *Spec Care Dent* **18**: 113–18.

40. Tenovuo J (2002). Clinical applications of antimicrobial host proteins lactoperoxidase, lysozyme and lactoferrin in xerostomia: efficacy and safety. *Oral Dis* **8**: 23–9.

41. Mulherin D, Ainsworth JR, Hamburger J, Situnayake D, Speculand B, Bowman SJ (2001). Survey of artificial tear and saliva usage among patients with Sjogren's syndrome. *Ann Rheum Dis* **60**: 1077–8.

42. Herod EL (1994). The use of milk as a saliva substitute. *J Public Health Dent* **54**: 184–9.

43. Kusler DL, Rambur BA (1992). Treatment for radiation-induced xerostomia. An innovative remedy. *Cancer Nurs* **15**: 191–5.

44. Walizer EM, Ephraim PM (1996). Double-blind cross-over controlled clinical trial of vegetable oil versus Xerolube for xerostomia: an expanded study abstract. *ORL Head Neck Nurs* **14**: 11–12.

45. Poland JM, Dugan M, Parashos P, Irick N, Dugan W, Tracey M (1987). Comparing Moi-Stir to lemon-glycerin swabs. *Am J Nurs* **87**: 422–4.

46. Abelson DC, Barton J, Mandel ID (1989). Effect of sorbitol sweetened breath mints on salivary flow and plaque pH in xerostomic subjects. *J Clin Den* **1**: 102–5.

47. Bjornstrom M, Axell T, Birkhed D (1990). Comparison between saliva stimulants and saliva substitutes in patients with symptoms related to dry mouth. A multi-centre study. *Swed Dent J* **14**: 153–61.

48. Stewart CM, Jones AC, Bates RE, Sandow P, Pink F, Stillwell J (1998). Comparison between saliva stimulants and a saliva substitute in patients with xerostomia and hyposalivation. *Spec Care Dentist* **18**: 142–8.

49. Aagaard A, Godiksen S, Teglers PT, Schiodt M, Glenert U (1992). Comparison between new saliva stimulants in patients with dry mouth: a placebo-controlled double-blind crossover study. *J Oral Pathol Med* **21**: 376–80.

50. Anneroth G, Nordenram G, Bengtsson S (1980). Effect of saliva stimulants (Hybrin® and malic acid) on cervical root surfaces in vitro. *Scand J Dent Res* **88**: 214–18.

51. Ferguson MM (1993). Pilocarpine and other cholinergic drugs in the management of salivary gland dysfunction. *Oral Surg Oral Med Oral Pathol* **75**: 186–91.

52. Fox PC, Atkinson JC, Macynski AA, Wolff A, Kung DS, Valdez IH *et al.* (1991). Pilocarpine treatment of salivary gland hypofunction and dry mouth (xerostomia). *Arch Intern Med* **151**: 1149–52.

53. Johnson JT, Ferretti GA, Nethery WJ, Valdez IH, Fox PC, Ng D *et al.* (1993). Oral pilocarpine for post-irradiation xerostomia in patients with head and neck cancer. *New Engl J Med* **329**: 390–5.

54. LeVeque FG, Montgomery M, Potter D, Zimmer MB, Rieke JW, Steiger BW *et al.* (1993). A multicentre, randomized, double-blind, placebo-controlled, dose-titration study of oral pilocarpine for treatment of radiation-induced xerostomia in head and neck cancer patients. *J Clin Oncol* **11**: 1124–31.

55. Davies AN, Singer J (1994). A comparison of artificial saliva and pilocarpine in radiation-induced xerostomia. *J Laryngol Otol* **108**: 663–5.

56. Rieke JW, Hafermann MD, Johnson JT, LeVeque FG, Iwamoto R, Steiger BW *et al.* (1995). Oral pilocarpine for radiation-induced xerostomia: integrated efficacy and safety results from two prospective randomized clinical trials. *Int J Radiat Oncol Biol Phys* **31**: 661–9.

57. Everett HC (1975). The use of bethanechol chloride with tricyclic antidepressants. *Am J Psychiatry* **132**: 1202–4.

58. Petrone D, Condemi JJ, Fife R, Gluck O, Cohen S, Dalgin P (2002). A double-blind, randomized, placebo-controlled study of cevimeline in Sjögren's syndrome patients with xerostomia and keratoconjunctivitis sicca. *Arthritis Rheum* **46**: 748–54.

59. Rydholm M, Strang P (1999). Acupuncture for patients in hospital-based home care suffering from xerostomia. *J Palliat Care* **15**: 20–3.

60. Johnstone PA, Niemtzow RC, Riffenburgh RH (2002). Acupuncture for xerostomia. *Cancer* **94**: 1151–6.

61. Blom M, Dawidson I, Angmar-Mansson B (1992). The effect of acupuncture on salivary flow rates in patients with xerostomia. *Oral Surg Oral Med Oral Pathol* **73**: 293–8.

62. Hamada T, Nakane T, Kimura T, Arisawa K, Yoneda K, Yamamoto T *et al.* (1999). Treatment of xerostomia with the bile secretion-stimulating drug anethole trithione: a clinical trial. *Am J Med Sci* **318**: 146–51.

63. Bagheri H, Schmitt L, Berlan M, Montastrue JL (1997). A comparative study of the effects of yohimbine and anetholtrithione on salivary secretion in depressed patients treated with psychotropic drugs. *Eur J Clin Pharmacol* **52**: 339–42.

64. Erlichman M (1990). Patient selection criteria for electrostimulation of salivary production in the treatment of xerostomia secondary to Sjögren's syndrome. *Health Technol Assess Rep* **8**: 1–7.

65. Sugano S, Takeyama I, Ogino S, Kenmochi M, Kaneko T (1996). Effectiveness of formula ophiopogoins in the treatment of xerostomia and pharyngoxerosis. *Acta Otolaryngol Suppl* **522**: 124–9.

Chapter 10

Taste disturbance

Carla Ripamonti and Fabio Fulfaro

Anatomy and physiology

The sensation of taste is mediated by the taste buds. There are about 10,000 taste buds, situated within the mucosa of the tongue, soft palate, uvula, pharynx, upper third of the oesophagus, epiglottis, larynx, lips and cheeks.[1,2]

The taste buds are connected to the oral cavity via the taste pores.[1] A protein ('gate-keeper') regulates the passage of saliva/tastants from the oral cavity, through the taste pore and into the taste bud. The taste buds consist of about 50 cells, including specialized gustatory cells. Gustatory cells have a microvillus (containing the taste receptor), which projects into the taste pore; gustatory cells also have a synapse, which connects to sensory nerve fibres. The gustatory cells are continuously being replaced (gustatory cells survive for ~ 10 days).

Each taste bud is innervated by about 50 nerve fibres, whilst each nerve fibre receives input from about five taste buds.[1] Taste information is transmitted via the V, VII, IX, and X cranial nerves to the nucleus of the tractus solitaris in the medulla, then onwards to the ventral posterior medial nucleus of the thalamus, and then onwards to the post central gyrus in the parietal lobe.

The four main taste qualities discernable by humans are bitter, salt, sour and sweet. However, other taste qualities are also discernible by humans, such as umami (glutamate-related taste quality).[1] Contrary to popular belief, the four main taste qualities are detectable in all areas of the tongue, rather than just in specific areas of the tongue.[1]

Genetic variation in taste is present within the population. Thus, people can be classified as 'non-tasters', 'tasters', or 'supertasters' according to their ability to recognize the bitterness of 6-n-propylthiouracil: 'non-tasters' cannot recognize the bitterness; 'tasters' can recognize the bitterness; 'supertasters' experience the most intense bitterness.[3]

It should be noted that taste refers to the specific perception of taste qualities (bitter, salt, sour, sugar), whilst flavour refers to the composite perceptions of taste, smell and oral somatosensory sensations (touch, temperature, nociception).[4]

Definitions

Taste disturbance occurs as a result of a reduction in taste sensation (hypogeusia), an absence of taste sensation (ageusia), or a distortion of normal taste sensation (dysgeusia).[5]

Table 10.1 Prevalence of taste disturbance in patients with advanced cancer

Study	Population	Prevalence (%)
Jobbins et al. 1992[6]	Hospice inpatient (N=197)	37
Davies and Kaur 1998[7]	Hospice inpatient (N=112)	40
Davies 2000[8]	Hospital support team (N=120)	44
Tranmer et al. 2003[9]	Hospital inpatient (N=66)	50

Epidemiology

Taste disturbance is relatively common in patients with advanced cancer (Table 10.1).[6–9] However, taste disturbance appears to be less common in patients with other advanced diseases.[9] Thus, Tranmer et al. reported a prevalence of only 19 per cent in a group of patients with chronic cardiac failure, chronic obstructive pulmonary disease, and cirrhosis.[9] However, the prevalence may be greater in other patient groups, e.g. patients with chronic renal failure.[10]

Aetiology

There are a variety of different causes of taste disturbance in the general population.[2] Figure 10.1 shows the common causes of taste disturbance in patients with cancer, although potentially any cause of taste disturbance could affect a patient with cancer.

Radiotherapy

Amongst the antineoplastic therapies, radiotherapy is the one most clearly linked to taste disturbance. Many patients have taste problems prior to head and neck radiotherapy, but almost all patients develop taste problems during head and neck radiotherapy.[11,12] Taste disturbance develops soon after the start of treatment (initial effect ~ at 1 week), and progresses during the early stage of treatment (maximum effect ~ 3–4 weeks).

In some cases, improvement in taste disturbance occurs within a few weeks/months of treatment. Nevertheless, in many cases, taste problems persist for a long time/indefinitely after treatment. For example, Maes et al. reported that 50 per cent of patients had subjective taste disturbance 12 months post radiotherapy.[12] Similarly, Mossman reported that some patients had objective taste disturbance 7 years post radiotherapy.[13]

Taste disturbance is the result of damage to the taste buds and/or salivary gland dysfunction. However, other factors may be relevant in some patients, such as the development of oral infection.[14] It is likely that the contribution of these factors varies from one individual to another. Thus, salivary gland dysfunction may be the most important factor in those patients that have persistent problems. (Salivary gland dysfunction is a long-term complication of head and neck radiotherapy).

It should be noted that some patients report that certain taste qualities are heightened following radiotherapy.[15]

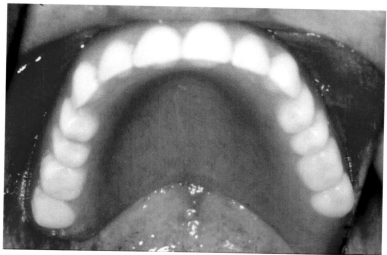

Plate 1 (a)   Denture in situ (no obvious oral pathology). (From M.P. Sweeney and J. Bagg (1997) *Making sense of the mouth*, Partnership in Oral Care, Glasgow. Reproduced with permission.) (See Chapter 2, Fig. 2.1(a))

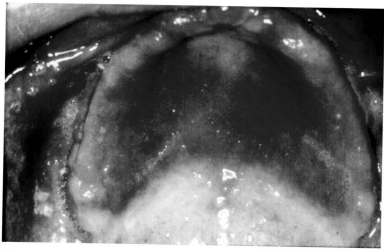

Plate 1 (b)   Denture removed revealing denture stomatitis. (From M.P. Sweeney and J. Bagg (1997) *Making sense of the mouth*, Partnership in Oral Care, Glasgow. Reproduced with permission.) (See Chapter 2, Fig. 2.1(b))

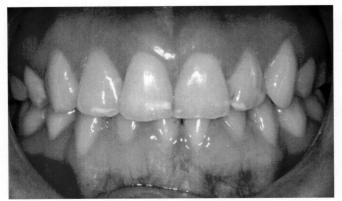

Plate 2   Normal appearance of gingiva/teeth. (Picture courtesy of J. Eveson.) (See Chapter 2, Fig. 2.3)

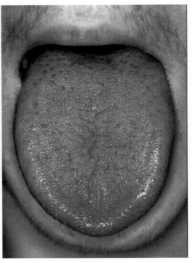

Plate 3   Normal appearance of tongue. (Picture courtesy of J. Eveson.) (See Chapter 2, Fig. 2.4.)

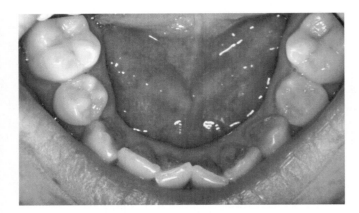

Plate 4   Normal appearance of floor of mouth. (Picture courtesy of J. Eveson.) (See Chapter 2, Fig. 2.5.)

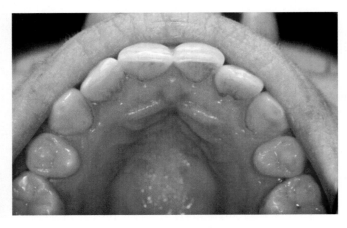

Plate 5   Normal appearance of roof of mouth. (Picture courtesy of J. Eveson.) (See Chapter 2, Fig. 2.6.)

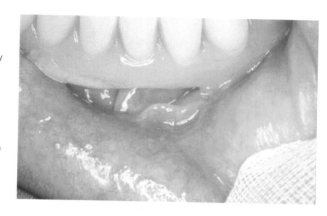

Plate 6 Denture granuloma/denture-induced hyperplasia. (From M.P. Sweeney and J. Bagg (1997) *Making sense of the mouth*, Partnership in Oral Care, Glasgow. Reproduced with permission.) (See Chapter 4, Fig. 4.3.)

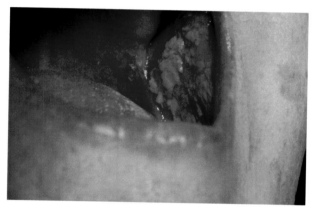

Plate 7 Pseudomembranous candidosis. (Picture courtesy of A. Davies.) (See Chapter 6, Fig. 6.1.)

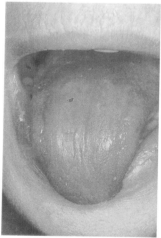

Plate 8 Erythematous candidosis. (Picture courtesy of A. Davies.) (See Chapter 6, Fig. 6.2.)

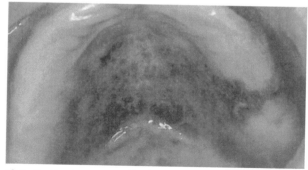

Plate 9 Denture stomatitis. (Picture courtesy of A. Davies.) (See Chapter 6, Fig. 6.3.)

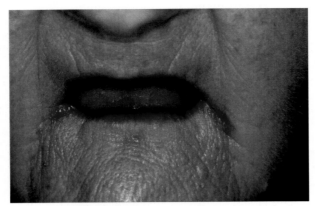

Plate 10 Angular cheilitis. (Picture courtesy of A. Davies.) (See Chapter 6, Fig. 6.4.)

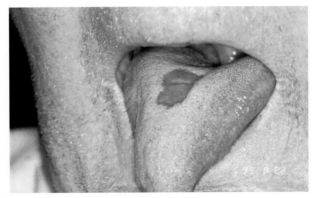

Plate 11 Median rhomboid glossitis. (Picture courtesy of J. Bagg.) (See Chapter 6, Fig. 6.5.)

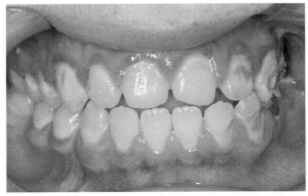

Plate 12 Early dental caries ("white spot lesion"). (Picture courtesy of G. Roberts.) (See Chapter 7, Fig. 7.1.)

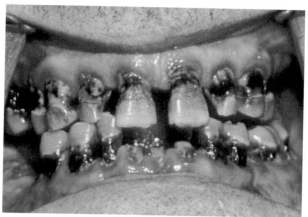

Plate 13 Advanced dental caries. (Picture courtesy of M. Chambers.) (See Chapter 7, Fig. 7.2.)

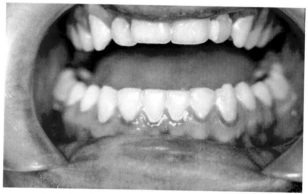

Plate 14 Plaque associated chronic marginal gingivitis. (Picture courtesy of Prof. David Wray.) (See Chapter 7, Fig. 7.4.)

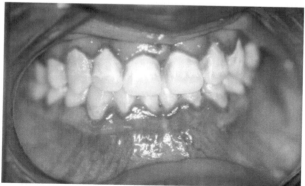

Plate 15 Acute necrotizing ulcerative gingivitis. (Picture courtesy of Dr Valli Meeks.) (See Chapter 7, Fig. 7.5.)

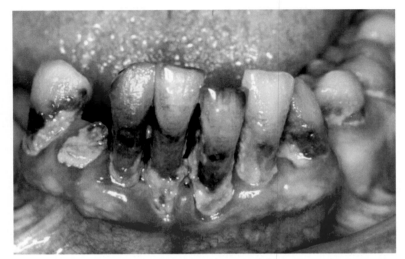

Plate 16 Adult periodontitis. (Picture courtesy of J. Bagg.) (See Chapter 7, Fig. 7.6.)

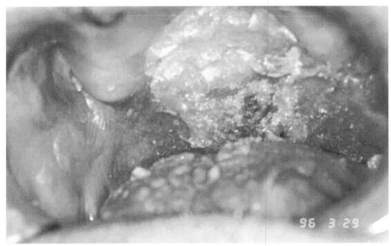

Plate 17 Staphylococcal mucositis. (Picture courtesy of M.P. Sweeney.) (See Chapter 7, Fig. 7.7.)

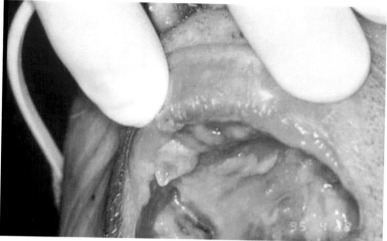

Plate 18 Staphylococcal mucositis. (From M.P. Sweeney and J. Bagg (1997) *Making sense of the mouth*, Partnership in Oral Care, Glasgow. Reproduced with permission.) (See Chapter 7, Fig. 7.8.)

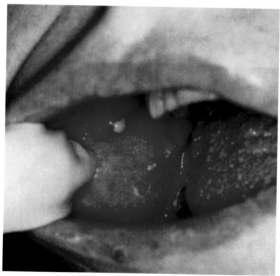

Plate 19 Acute bacterial parotitis (pus draining from parotid duct). (From W.R. Tyldesley and A. Field (1993) *Oral medicine*, 4th edn, Oxford University Press, Oxford. Reproduced with permission.) (See Chapter 7, Fig. 7.9.)

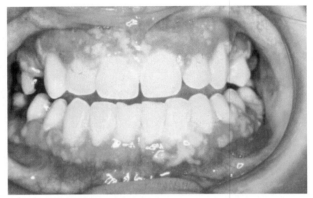

Plate 20 Primary herpes simplex virus infection (primary herpetic gingivostomatitis). (From M.P. Sweeney and J. Bagg (1997) *Making sense of the mouth*, Partnership in Oral Care, Glasgow. Reproduced with permission.) (See Chapter 8, Fig. 8.1.)

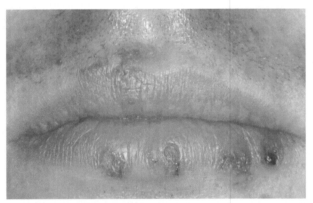

Plate 21 Secondary herpes simplex virus infection in immunocompetent patient (herpes labialis). (Picture courtesy of J. Eveson.) (See Chapter 8, Fig. 8.2.)

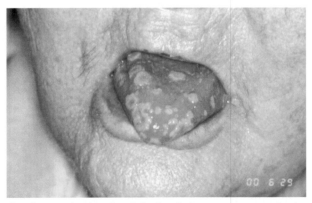

Plate 22 Secondary herpes simplex virus infection in immunocompromised patient. (Picture courtesy of M.P. Sweeney.) (See Chapter 8, Fig. 8.3.)

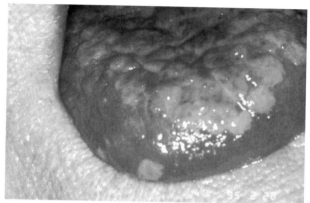

Plate 23 Secondary herpes simplex virus infection in immunocompromised patient. (From M.P. Sweeney and J. Bagg (1997) *Making sense of the mouth*, Partnership in Oral Care, Glasgow. Reproduced with permission.) (See Chapter 8, Fig. 8.4.)

Plate 24 (a) Secondary varicella zoster (facial component). (From M.P. Sweeney and J. Bagg (1997) *Making sense of the mouth*, Partnership in Oral Care, Glasgow. Reproduced with permission.) (See Chapter 8, Fig. 8.5(a).)

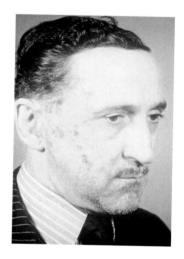

(b) Secondary varicella zoster (oral component). (From M.P. Sweeney and J. Bagg (1997) *Making sense of the mouth*, Partnership in Oral Care, Glasgow. Reproduced with permission.) (See Chapter 8, Fig. 8.5(b).)

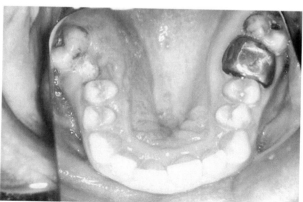

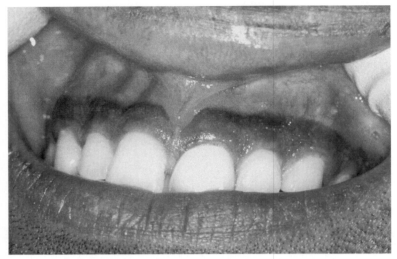

Plate 25   Racial pigmentation. (Picture courtesy of J. Eveson.) (See Chapter 13, Fig. 13.1.)

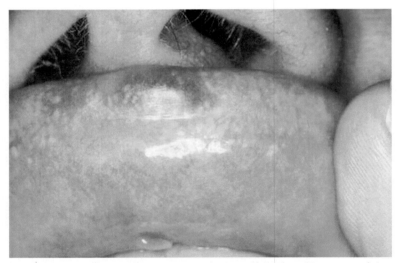

Plate 26   Oral varicosity. (From M.P. Sweeney and J. Bagg (1997) *Making sense of the mouth*, Partnership in Oral Care, Glasgow. Reproduced with permission.) (See Chapter 13, Fig. 13.2.)

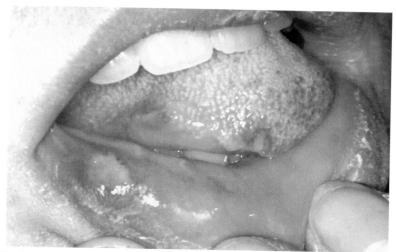

Plate 27 Recurrent minor aphthous ulceration. (Picture courtesy of J. Eveson.) (See Chapter 13, Fig. 13.3.)

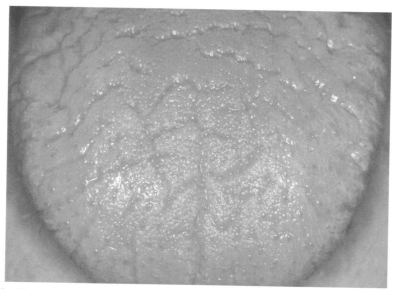

Plate 28 Fissured tongue. (Picture courtesy of J. Eveson.) (See Chapter 13, Fig. 13.4.)

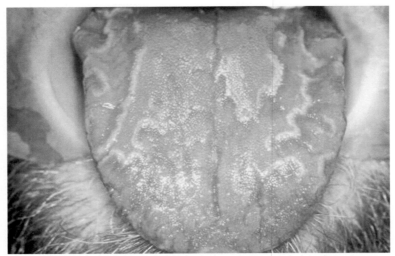

Plate 29 Geographic tongue. (From M.P. Sweeney and J. Bagg (1997) *Making sense of the mouth*, Partnership in Oral Care, Glasgow. Reproduced with permission.) (See Chapter 13, Fig. 13.5.)

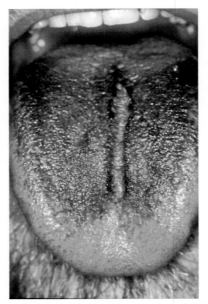

Plate 30 Black hairy tongue. (From M.P. Sweeney and J. Bagg (1997) *Making sense of the mouth*, Partnership in Oral Care, Glasgow. Reproduced with permission.) (See Chapter 13, Fig. 13.6.)

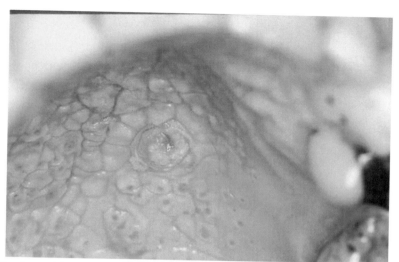

Plate 31   Stomatitis nicotina. (From M.P. Sweeney and J. Bagg (1997) *Making sense of the mouth*, Partnership in Oral Care, Glasgow. Reproduced with permission.) (See Chapter 13, Fig. 13.7.)

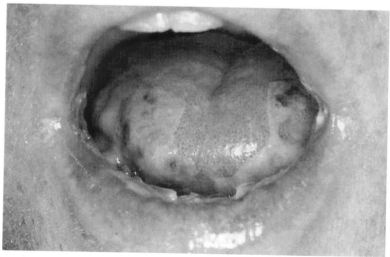

Plate 32   Chemotherapy-induced mucositis. (Picture courtesy of M. Chambers.) (See Chapter 15, Fig. 15.1.)

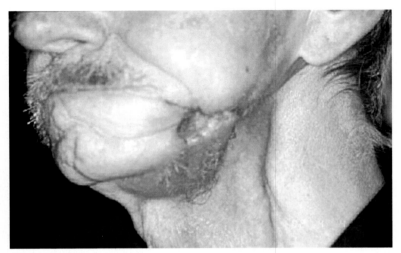

Plate 33 Osteoradionecrosis. (Picture courtesy of M.P. Sweeney.) (See Chapter 15, Fig. 15.2.)

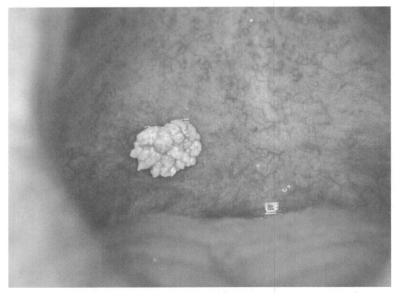

Plate 34 Oral wart. (Picture courtesy of J. Eveson.) (See Chapter 16, Fig. 16.2.)

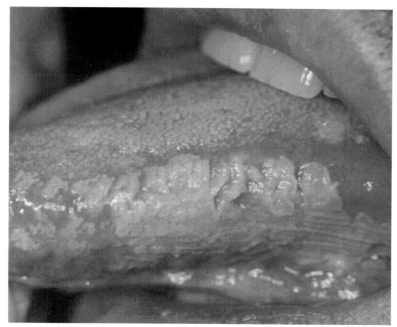

Plate 35 Oral hairy leukoplakia. (Picture courtesy of Dr Valli Meeks.) (See Chapter 16, Fig. 16.3.)

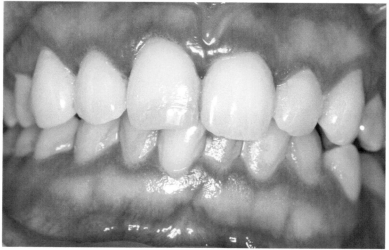

Plate 36 Linear gingival erythema. (Picture courtesy of J. Eveson.) (See Chapter 16, Fig. 16.4.)

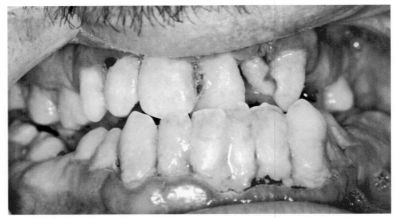

Plate 37 Necrotizing ulcerative periodontitis. (Picture courtesy of Dr Jane Luker.) (See Chapter 16, Fig. 16.5.)

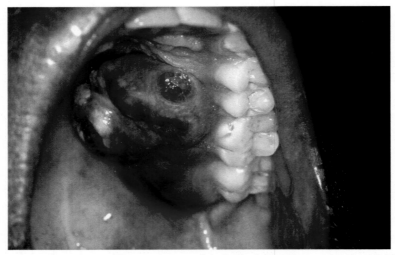

Plate 38 Kaposi's sarcoma. (Picture courtesy of A. Davies.) (See Chapter 16, Fig. 16.6.)

- **Cancer-related**
  - Specific effect: damage of taste buds/cranial nerves (V, VII, IX, X)/ central nervous system
  - Non-specific effect

- **Cancer treatment-related**
  - Local surgery
  - Local radiotherapy
  - Systemic chemotherapy

- **Oral problems**
  - Salivary gland dysfunction
  - Poor oral hygiene
  - Oral infections
  - Other oral pathology
  - Dental prosthesis ('denture')

- **Neurological problems**
  - Damage of cranial nerves (V, VII, IX, X)
  - Damage of central nervous system

- **Metabolic problems**
  - Malnutrition
  - Zinc deficiency
  - Renal dysfunction
  - Liver dysfunction
  - Endocrine dysfunction

- **Miscellaneous**
  - Ageing
  - Menopause
  - Drug treatment
  - Smoking
  - Other chronic diseases

Fig. 10.1 Aetiology of taste disturbance in patients with cancer.

Chemotherapy

Antineoplastic drugs that have been associated with taste changes include bleomycin, carboplatin, cisplatin, cyclophosphamide, doxorubicin, 5-fluorouracil, gemcitabine, levamisole and methotrexate.[16] In most cases there is little data about the nature of the taste disturbance with these drugs. However, Wickham *et al.* reported that the metallic taste induced by cisplatin may last from a few hours to 3 weeks.[16]

Drug therapy

A variety of different drugs have been reported to cause taste disturbance.[2] However, certain classes of drug seem to be particularly problematic, including anti-inflammatory agents and antimicrobial agents.[17] Some drugs cause taste disturbance per se, whilst others cause it through indirect mechanisms, e.g. induction of salivary gland dysfunction.

Zinc deficiency

Zinc depletion has been linked to impaired taste function in pregnant women, in the elderly, in patients with cancer[18] and in patients with other chronic diseases.[10] Furthermore, drugs with sulphydryl groups, which chelate zinc, are associated with taste disturbance (e.g. D-penicillamine).

The specific role of zinc in the control of taste is unknown.[19] Zinc is the co-factor for alkaline phosphatase, the most abundant enzyme in the taste bud membrane. Furthermore zinc, and other metals, control the conformation of the protein ('gate-keeper') that regulates the passage of tastants through the taste bud pore.

Clinical features

Taste disturbance can lead to physical, psychological, and social problems, which, in turn, can lead to deterioration in quality of life. Figure 10.2 shows quotations from patients with taste disturbance, which demonstrate the wide-ranging problems that may occur.[20]

Patients may complain of a single taste problem (e.g. ageusia for all foods), or a combination of taste problems (e.g. hypogeusia for some foods, dysgeusia for other foods). For example, in a study involving patients with advanced cancer and taste disturbance, 40 per cent reported ageusia, 31 per cent reported hypogeusia, and 53 per cent reported dysgeusia.[7] Patients with dysgeusia may report a variety of different sensations, but invariably report that food tastes unpleasant.[21]

Table 1.4 shows the severity of taste problems in a group of patients with advanced cancer.[8] It can be seen that the majority (70 per cent) of patients reported that their taste disturbance was 'moderate', 'severe', or 'very severe'. Table 1.5 shows the distress caused by taste problems in the same group of patients with advanced cancer.[8] It can be seen that the majority (51 per cent) of patients reported that their taste disturbance caused significant distress. Other studies have reported similar results.[7]

Quote A

'Sweet food had a bad taste, strong food was burning and tingling on the tongue. Fluids with carbonic acid felt like hydrochloric acid.'

Quote B

'We were to celebrate my birthday and I had helped to prepare salmon and looked forward to have dinner with the family. The taste alteration was incredible, the food tasted of absolutely nothing or possibly of wheat flour; I was disappointed and depressed and felt sorry for myself, I couldn't feel or share happiness with my family during that occasion.'

Quote C

'I wanted to surprise my family with a nice meal, with my speciality which is salty herring. Normally, I am very proud of it but I totally failed with the seasoning as I did not feel the taste, I used far too much salt, the meal was uneatable. I was so embarrassed.'

Fig. 10.2 Quotations from patients with taste disturbance.[20]

Impairment of taste may be associated with anorexia[22] and also weight loss.[18] However, the association is much stronger for anorexia, than for weight loss. Impairment of taste may affect other aspects of gastrointestinal function, i.e. reduce salivary gland secretion, reduce intestinal motility.[5]

Investigations

It is uncommon for patients to report taste disturbance.[5] The reasons why patients do not report taste disturbance are unknown. However, patients may not report a symptom if: (a) they perceive the symptom to be inevitable; (b) they perceive there is no treatment for the symptom; (c) they sense that healthcare professionals perceive the symptom to be unimportant; and/or (d) other symptoms predominate.[23] Thus, it is important that patients are specifically asked about taste disturbance.

The assessment of taste disturbance involves taking a history, performing an examination, and undertaking appropriate investigations.[24] It is not necessary to obtain an objective assessment of the problem (i.e. measure taste acuity). The assessment of oral problems is discussed in detail in Chapter 2.

Taste acuity may be assessed using the standard three-stimulus drop technique to measure the detection and recognition thresholds for the four main taste qualities (bitter, salt, sour, sweet).[25] The detection threshold is the lowest concentration of solute that the subject distinguishes as being different from water, whereas the recognition threshold is the lowest concentration of solute that the subject recognizes correctly.

Management

The management of taste disturbance involves:

- Treatment of the underlying cause
- Dietary therapy
- Zinc therapy; and/or
- Other therapies.

Treatment of the underlying cause

In some cases it may be possible to treat the underlying cause of the taste disturbance, e.g. salivary gland dysfunction. Indeed, studies have shown that saliva stimulants improve both the xerostomia, and the associated taste disturbance.[26] (In contrast, studies have shown that saliva substitutes only improve the xerostomia.[26]) Nevertheless, in many cases, it is not possible to identify and/or treat the underlying cause of the taste disturbance.

Dietary therapy

Dietary therapy involves: (a) utilization of foods that taste 'good'; (b) avoidance of foods that taste 'bad'; (c) enhancing the taste of the food (using salt, sugar and other flavourings); and (d) addressing the presentation, smell, consistency and temperature of the food.[27,28] Ideally, a dietician should review all patients with taste disturbance, since dietary therapy requires an individualized approach.[29]

Zinc therapy

The most studied therapy in patients with taste disturbance is oral zinc. Zinc has been used to treat taste disturbance in a number of different clinical settings. Table 10.2 shows data from clinical studies involving patients with cancer.[11,30–32] All of these studies involved patients with radiotherapy-related taste problems. Thus, the results may not be generalizable to patients with other cancer-related taste problems.

It was found that zinc given during radiotherapy limited the degree of objective taste disturbance, and also shortened the recovery time of both subjective and objective taste disturbance.[30,32] It should be noted that zinc salts are considered to be radioprotectors.[33] Similarly, it was found that zinc given post radiotherapy improved both

Table 10.2 Studies of zinc administration in patients with cancer

Study	Design	Regimen	Outcomes
Mossman and Henkin 1978[11]	Case series N = 7; patients with taste disturbance post head and neck radiotherapy	Variable 25 or 100 mg/day zinc for 2–6 months	Improvement in objective taste disturbance Improvement in anorexia (and weight gain)
Silverman et al. 1983[30]	Randomized controlled trial vs placebo N = 19; patients pre head and neck radiotherapy	18 mg qds zinc for duration of radiotherapy	No difference in objective taste disturbance during radiotherapy between groups Earlier recovery of subjective taste disturbance in treatment group (64% vs 22% patients at 3 weeks post treatment).
Silverman et al. 1984[31]	Case series N = 30; patients with taste disturbance post head and neck radiotherapy	Variable 100–150 mg/day zinc for at least 1 month	Improvement in subjective taste disturbance (37% of patients)
Ripamonti et al. 1998[32]	Randomized controlled trial vs placebo N = 18; patients with taste disturbance during head and neck radiotherapy	45 mg tds zinc sulphate from onset of subjective taste disturbance until 1 month post radiotherapy	Less objective taste disturbance during radiotherapy in treatment group Earlier recovery of objective taste disturbance in treatment group

subjective and objective taste disturbance.[11,31] However, Silverman *et al.* reported that only 37 per cent of patients improved subjectively with zinc supplements.[31]

Studies in other patient groups have produced conflicting results. For example, some large studies involving patients with idiopathic/mixed aetiology taste disturbance have not reported a positive effect.[34,35] In contrast, for example, some smaller studies involving patients with renal disease have reported a positive effect (i.e. objective improvement).[10,36] Thus, it may be that zinc is effective for some, but not all, causes of taste disturbance.

The aforementioned studies suggest that zinc salts are generally well tolerated. (Zinc salts can cause dyspepsia, and abdominal pain.) Thus, on the basis of the available evidence, it would seem appropriate to offer patients with taste disturbance a trial of an oral zinc salt (e.g. zinc sulphate).

Other treatments

Other treatments that have been used to treat taste disturbance include copper,[37] nickel,[38] corticosteroids[27] and various complementary therapies. However, the evidence for their efficacy/tolerability is weak.

References

1. Ganong WF (2003). *Review of Medical Physiology,* 21st edn, pp. 191–4. New York: Lange Medical Books.
2. Schiffman SS (1983). Taste and smell in disease (first of two parts). *New Engl J Med* **308**: 1275–9.
3. Bartoshuk LM (2000). Comparing sensory experiences across individuals: recent psychophysical advances illuminate genetic variation in taste perception. *Chem Senses* **25**: 447–60.
4. Duffy VB, Fast K, Lucchina LA, Bartoshuk LM (2002). Oral sensation and cancer. In AM Berger, RK Portenoy, DE Weissman (ed.) *Principles and Practice of Palliative Care and Supportive Oncology*, 2nd edn, pp. 178–93. Philadelphia: Lippincott Williams & Wilkins.
5. De Conno F, Sbanotto A, Ripamonti C, Ventafridda V (2003). Mouth Care. In D Doyle, G Hanks, N Cherny, K Calman (ed.) *Oxford Textbook of Palliative Medicine*, 3rd edn, pp. 673–87. Oxford: Oxford University Press.
6. Jobbins J, Bagg J, Finlay IG, Addy M, Newcombe RG (1992). Oral and dental disease in terminally ill cancer patients. *BMJ* **304**: 1612.
7. Davies AN, Kaur K (1998). Taste problems in patients with advanced cancer. *Palliat Med* **12**: 482–3.
8. Davies ANT (2000). An investigation into the relationship between salivary gland hypofunction and oral health problems in patients with advanced cancer. Dissertation. King's College: University of London.
9. Tranmer JE, Heyland D, Dudgeon D, Groll D, Squires-Graham M, Coulson K (2003). Measuring the symptom experience of seriously ill cancer and noncancer hospitalized patients near the end of life with the Memorial Symptom Assessment Scale. *J Pain Symptom Manage* **25**: 420–9.
10. Atkin-Thor E, Goddard BW, O'Nion J, Stephen RL, Kolff WJ (1978). Hypogeusia and zinc depletion in chronic dialysis patients. *Am J Clin Nutr* **31**: 1948–51.

11. Mossman KL, Henkin RI (1978). Radiation-induced changes in taste acuity in cancer patients. *Int J Radiat Oncol Biol Phys* **4**: 663–70.

12. Maes A, Huygh I, Weltens C, Vandevelde G, Delaere P, Evers G *et al.* (2002). De Gustibus: time scale of loss and recovery of tastes caused by radiotherapy. *Radiother Oncol* **63**: 195–201.

13. Mossman KL, Shatzman AR, Chencharick JD (1982). Long-term effects of radiotherapy on taste and salivary function in man. *Int J Radiat Oncol Biol Phys* **8**: 991–7.

14. Fernando IN, Patel T, Billingham L, Hammond C, Hallmark S, Glaholm J *et al.* (1995). The effect of head and neck irradiation on taste dysfunction: a prospective study. *Clin Oncol (R Coll Radiol)* **7**: 173–8.

15. Bonanni G, Perazzi F (1965). Il comportamento della sensibilita' gustativa in pazienti sottoposti a trattamento radiologico con alte energie per tumori del cavo orale. *Nunt Radiol* **31**: 383–97.

16. Wickham RS, Rehwaldt M, Kefer C, Shott S, Abbas K, Glynn-Tucker E *et al.* (1999). Taste changes experienced by patients receiving chemotherapy. *Oncol Nurs Forum* **26**: 697–706.

17. Schiffman SS, Zervakis J, Westall HL, Graham BG, Metz A, Bennett JL *et al.* (2000). Effect of antimicrobial and anti-inflammatory medications on the sense of taste. *Physiol Behav* **69**: 413–24.

18. DeWys WD, Walters K (1975). Abnormalities of taste sensation in cancer patients. *Cancer* **36**: 1888–96.

19. Ripamonti C, Fulfaro F (1998). Taste alterations in cancer patients. *J Pain Symptom Manage* **16**: 349–51.

20. Rydholm M, Strang P (2002). Physical and psychosocial impact of xerostomia in palliative cancer care: a qualitative interview study. *Int J Palliat Nurs* **8**: 318–23.

21. Shapiro SL (1974). Abnormalities of taste. *Eye Ear Nose Throat Mon* **53**: 293–6.

22. Stubbs L (1989). Taste changes in cancer patients. *Nurs Times* **18**: 49–50.

23. Shorthose K, Davies AN (2003). Symptom prevalence in palliative care. *Palliat Med* **17**: 73–4.

24. Birnbaum W, Dunne SM (2000). *Oral Diagnosis: the clinician's guide*. Oxford: Wright.

25. Henkin RI, Schechter PJ, Hoye R, Mattern CF (1971). Idiopathic hypogeusia with dysgeusia, hyposmia and dysosmia. A new syndrome. *J Am Med Assoc* **217**: 434–40.

26. Davies AN, Singer J (1994). A comparison of artificial saliva and pilocarpine in radiation-induced xerostomia. *J Laryngol Otol* **108**: 663–5.

27. Twycross RG, Lack SA (1986). Taste changes. In *Control of Alimentary Symptoms in Far Advanced Cancer*, pp. 57–65. Edinburgh: Churchill Livingstone.

28. Komurcu S, Nelson KA, Walsh D (2000). The gastrointestinal symptoms of advanced cancer. *Support Care Cancer* **9**: 32–9.

29. Davidson I, Richardson R (2003). Dietary and nutritional aspects of palliative medicine. In D Doyle, G Hanks, N Cherny, K Calman (ed.) *Oxford Textbook of Palliative Medicine*, 3rd edn, pp. 546–52. Oxford: Oxford University Press.

30. Silverman JE, Weber CW, Silverman S Jr, Coulthard SL, Manning MR (1983). Zinc supplementation and taste in head and neck cancer patients undergoing radiation therapy. *J Oral Med* **38**: 14–16.

31. Silverman S Jr, Thompson JS (1984). Serum zinc and copper in oral/oropharyngeal carcinoma. A study of seventy-five patients. *Oral Surg Oral Med Oral Pathol* **57**: 34–6.

32. Ripamonti C, Zecca E, Brunelli C, Fulfaro F, Villa S, Balzarini A *et al.* (1998). A randomized, controlled clinical trial to evaluate the effects of zinc sulfate on cancer patients with taste alterations caused by head and neck irradiation. *Cancer* **82**: 1938–45.

33. Floersheim GL, Bieri A (1990). Further studies on selective radioprotection by organic zinc salts and synergism of zinc aspartate with WR 2721. *Br J Radiol* **63**: 468–75.

34. Henkin RI, Schecter PJ, Friedewald WT, Demets DL, Raff M (1976). A double blind study of the effects of zinc sulfate on taste and smell dysfunction. *Am J Med Sci* **272**: 285–99.

35. Sakai F, Yoshida S, Endo S, Tomita H (2002). Double-blind, placebo-controlled trial of zinc picolinate for taste disorders. *Acta Otolaryngol Suppl (Stockh)* **546**: 129–33.

36. Mahajan SK, Prasad AS, Lambujon J, Abbasi AA, Briggs WA, McDonald FD (1980). Improvement of uremic hypogeusia by zinc: a double-blind study. *Am J Clin Nutr* **33**: 1517–21.

37. Henkin RI, Keiser HR, Jafee IA, Sternlieb I, Scheinberg IH (1967). Decreased taste sensitivity after D-penicillamine reversed by copper administration. *Lancet* **2**: 1268–71.

38. Henkin RI, Bradley DF (1970). Hypogeusia corrected by Ni++ and Zn++. *Life Sci II* **9**: 701–9.

Chapter 11

Halitosis

Kate Shorthose and Andrew Davies

Definition

Halitosis has been defined as 'offensive odours from the mouth or hollow cavities such as the nose, sinuses, and pharynx'.[1] Other terms used to describe this condition include oral malodour, foetor oris ('stench of the mouth'), foetor ex ore ('stench from the mouth'), and 'bad breath'.[2]

Epidemiology

Halitosis is a problem that everyone has from time to time, but that some people have on a more regular basis.[3] The reported prevalence of chronic subjective halitosis varies between 25–50 per cent.[4] However, the reported prevalence of chronic objective halitosis varies between 2.4–30 per cent.[5] It should be noted that the lower figure reflects severe halitosis, whilst the upper figure reflects mild to moderate halitosis.

Gordon *et al.* reported that 48 per cent of hospice patients complained of 'bad breath'.[6] However, it would appear that there are no other data on the prevalence of halitosis in the palliative care setting. Nevertheless, it is generally accepted that halitosis is a problem in this area.[6]

Aetiology

An aetiological classification of halitosis is shown in Fig. 11.1.[7]

Physiological halitosis is the commonest type in the general population, and probably the commonest type of halitosis in the palliative care setting. Patients with physiological halitosis do not have an underlying disease causing the oral malodour:[7] the cause of physiological halitosis is the bacterial putrefaction of food debris, epithelial cells, blood cells and saliva within the oral cavity.[5,8]

The process of putrefaction involves the conversion of proteins, polypeptides, and amino acids into volatile sulphur compounds (e.g. hydrogen sulphide, methyl mercaptan), and volatile non-sulphur compounds (e.g. diamines, volatile fatty acids).[8] A variety of bacterial species have been implicated in the process, especially the anaerobic, Gram-negative bacterial species.[5] The process of putrefaction can occur anywhere within the oral cavity, but occurs mainly on the posterior part of the dorsum of the tongue.

- **Genuine halitosis** – malodour present

  - *Physiological halitosis* – no underlying disease present

  - *Pathological halitosis* – underlying disease present

    1 Oral causes

    2 Extra-oral causes:

      (a) Disease of the upper respiratory tract

      (b) Disease of the lower respiratory tract

      (c) Disease of the gastrointestinal tract

      (d) Systemic metabolic problems

- **Pseudohalitosis** – malodour not present

- **Halitophobia** – malodour not present

Fig. 11.1 Aetiology of halitosis.[7]

Patients with pathological halitosis have an underlying disease causing the oral malodour.[7] The underlying disease may be an infection, inflammation, or malignancy. In most (~90 per cent) cases, the source of the malodour is the oral cavity, but other potential sources include the upper respiratory tract (nose, sinuses), the lower respiratory tract, the gastrointestinal tract, or a systemic metabolic problem. Oral causes of malodour include salivary gland dysfunction, as well as infection and malignancy. Systemic metabolic causes of malodour include renal impairment, liver impairment, malnutrition, and diabetes mellitus (ketoacidosis).

Pseudohalitosis and halitophobia are non-organic disorders. Patients with these conditions believe that they have oral malodour, although there is no objective evidence to support this belief.[7] Patients with pseudohalitosis respond to educational interventions. However, patients with halitophobia do not respond to educational interventions, and require formal psychological/psychiatric therapy.[7] Halitophobia may occur in isolation, or in combination with other psychological/psychiatric problems.[8]

Clinical features

Halitosis is a major cause of morbidity within the general population, and also within the palliative care population.[6]

The patient may, or may not, be aware of the fact that they have halitosis: the patient may be unaware that they have halitosis, because they have developed an olfactory disturbance[4] or they have developed tolerance to the malodour (habituation).[9] It should be noted that some patients complain of taste disturbance ('bad taste'), whilst others complain of symptoms relating to the underlying cause of the halitosis.[4]

Even if the patient is aware that they have halitosis, it is unusual for them to complain about the halitosis. There are a number of explanations for this phenomenon: (a) the patient is embarrassed to admit that they have halitosis; (b) they perceive the symptom to be inevitable; (c) they perceive there is no treatment for the symptom; (d) they sense that healthcare professionals perceive the symptom to be unimportant; and/or (e) other symptoms/problems predominate.[10]

Halitosis can have profound psychological and social effects.[4] Patients may be embarrassed by the malodour, and so avoid intimate contact with family and friends. Similarly, family and friends may find it difficult to tolerate the malodour, and so avoid contact with the patient. Moreover, healthcare professionals may limit their interactions with the patient. Thus, a barrier develops between the patient and their carers, which impacts on every aspect of daily life/routine care. Patients may become depressed by the reaction of the carers, and the carers become distressed by their reaction to the patient.

Investigations

The assessment of a patient with halitosis involves taking a history, performing an examination, and use of appropriate investigations (to determine the aetiology of the halitosis).

The assessment of the oral malodour involves:[7]

- ◆ Organoleptic measurement
- ◆ Gas chromatography
- ◆ Sulphide monitoring

Organoleptic measurement

Organoleptic measurement is the usual method of assessing halitosis. It consists of the investigator smelling the patient's breath, and assigning it an 'organoleptic score' (Table 11.1). Specific protocols have been developed to standardize the assessment: the protocol specifies the physical set up, pre-test instructions for the patient (e.g. avoidance of certain foods), and pre-test instructions for the investigator (e.g. avoidance of scented products).[7]

It is often possible to distinguish the source of the malodour by smelling the air expired from the nose, as well as from the mouth. For example, if the breath expired from the nose is more offensive than the breath from the mouth, then this suggests that

Table 11.1 Organoleptic scoring scale[7]

Category	Description
0 Absence of odour	Odour cannot be detected
1 Questionable odour	Odour is detectable, although the examiner could not recognize it as malodour
2 Slight malodour	Odour is deemed to exceed the threshold of malodour recognition
3 Moderate malodour	Malodour is definitely detected
4 Strong malodour	Strong malodour is detected, but can be tolerated by examiner
5 Severe malodour	Overwhelming malodour is detected and cannot be tolerated by examiner (examiner instinctively averts the nose)

the source of the malodour is the nose/sinuses, rather than the mouth (and vice versa).[8] If the breath expired from the nose is as offensive as the breath expired from the mouth, then this suggests that the source of the malodour is the lower respiratory tract, the gastrointestinal tract, or a systemic metabolic problem.[8]

Gas chromatography

Gas chromatography is the 'gold standard' method for assessing halitosis. The equipment is not portable, or easy to use, which means that this method is not suitable for routine clinical use.

Sulphide monitoring

Sulphide monitoring is a reasonably standard method for assessing halitosis. The equipment is portable, and easy to use, which means that this method is suitable for routine clinical use. However, the portable monitors are not particularly sensitive (i.e. certain relevant compounds are not detected), or particularly specific (i.e. certain non-relevant compound are detected).[4]

Management

The management of the halitosis depends on the aetiology of the halitosis.[7] For example, patients with pathological halitosis require treatment for the underlying disease process. Similarly, patients with pseudohalitosis require educational interventions, and patients with halitophobia require psychological/psychiatric interventions.

The management of physiological halitosis includes:[11]

◆ Dietary modification

◆ Smoking cessation

◆ Measures to reduce bacterial numbers

◆ Measures to reduce bacterial substrates

- Measures to convert volatile sulphur compounds to non-volatile compounds
- Use of masking agents
- Use of 'natural products'.

In general, diet is not a major causative factor. However, it would seem appropriate to avoid foods that are associated with oral malodour, e.g. garlic, onions.[12]

Maintenance of oral hygiene is essential for improving halitosis: teeth cleaning, interdental cleaning, and oral rinsing all improve oral malodour by reducing bacterial numbers, and by reducing the amount of substrate available to the bacteria.[11] Moreover, many toothpastes contain antibacterial agents, and/or other relevant agents. For example, baking soda (sodium bicarbonate) is antibacterial, and can also convert volatile sulphur compounds to non-volatile compounds. Some patients may also benefit from periodontal treatment to reduce periodontal bacterial numbers (i.e. scaling, root planing).

As discussed above, the tongue is the main source of the malodour. Tongue cleaning will improve halitosis by reducing bacterial numbers, and by reducing the amount of substrate available to the bacteria.[7,11] The tongue can be cleaned with an ordinary toothbrush, a paediatric toothbrush, a tongue brush, or a 'tongue scraper' (Fig. 11.2). The aim of cleaning is to remove the coating on the tongue, without damaging the mucosa of the tongue. Thus, cleaning should be performed very gently, and should be discontinued once the coating has been removed/becomes difficult to remove.

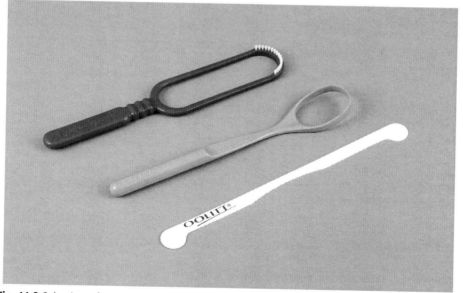

Fig. 11.2 Selection of tongue cleaners.

It is important to clean as far back as possible, since the putrefaction occurs mainly on the posterior part of the tongue.

Mechanical methods of reducing bacterial numbers can be supplemented with chemical methods of reducing bacterial numbers.[11] Chlorhexidine is very effective, but is often associated with side-effects (see Chapter 3). Other antibacterial agents that have been used to treat halitosis, include cetylpyridinium chloride, essential oils (Listerine®), hydrogen peroxide, and triclosan. These agents have been incorporated into conventional mouthwashes, 'two-phase' mouthwashes, toothpastes and chewing gum. Two-phase mouthwashes consist of an aqueous component that contains anti-bacterial agents, and an oil component that acts as a bacterial 'trap' (the bacteria adhere to the oil).

A novel way of treating halitosis is to convert the volatile sulphur compounds into non-volatile (non-odorous) compounds.[11] Various agents can be used, including zinc salts, tin salts, baking soda and chlorine dioxide. Zinc salts, particularly zinc chloride, have been incorporated into a range of mouthwashes, toothpastes and chewing gum.

In most cases, a combination of treatments is required to control the halitosis (mechanical methods, chemical methods). It should be noted that studies suggest that mouthwashes are more effective than toothpastes,[5] and that products with multiple agents are more effective than products with single agents.[11]

A variety of commercial products have been developed to counteract the malodour including mints, chewing gum and deodorant-type mouthwashes/sprays. However, these products mask the problem, rather than treat the problem. Moreover, these products tend to have a very short duration of action. In addition, a variety of 'natural products' have been used to treat halitosis, including herbs (various), tea (black) and an extract of Salvadora persica ('the toothbrush tree').

References

1. Nachnani S, Clark GT (1997). Halitosis: a breath of fresh air. *Clin Infect Dis* **25**, Suppl 2: S218–19.
2. Spouge JD (1964). Halitosis, A review of its causes and treatment. *Dent Pract Dent Rec* **14**: 307–17.
3. Scully C, Porter S, Greenman J (1994). What to do about halitosis. *BMJ* **308**: 217–18.
4. Bosy A (1997). Oral malodor: philosophical and practical aspects. *J Can Dent Assoc* **63**: 196–201.
5. Loesche WJ, Kazor C (2002). Microbiology and treatment of halitosis. *Periodontol 2000* **28**: 256–79.
6. Gordon SR, Berkey DB, Call RL (1985). Dental need among hospice patients in Colorado: a pilot study. *Gerodontics* **1**: 125–9.
7. Yaegaki K, Coil JM (2000). Examination, classification, and treatment of halitosis; clinical perspectives. *J Can Dent Assoc* **66**: 257–61.
8. Ayers KM, Colquhoun AN (1998). Halitosis: causes, diagnosis, and treatment. *N Z Dent J* **94**: 156–60.

9. Rosenberg M, Kozlovsky A, Gelernter I, Cherniak O, Gabbay J, Baht R *et al.* (1995). Self-estimation of oral malodor. *J Dent Res* **74**: 1577–82.

10. Shorthose K, Davies AN (2003). Symptom prevalence in palliative care. *Palliat Med* **17**: 723–4.

11. Quirynen M, Zhao H, van Steenberghe D (2002). Review of the treatment strategies for oral malodour. *Clin Oral Investig* **6**: 1–10.

12. De Conno F, Sbanotto A, Ripamonti C, Ventafridda V (2003). Mouth Care. In D Doyle, G Hanks, N Cherny, K Calman (ed.) *Oxford Textbook of Palliative Medicine*, 3rd edn, pp. 673–87. Oxford: Oxford University Press.

Chapter 12

Oral pain

John Meechan

Epidemiology

Oral discomfort/pain is relatively common in patients receiving specialist palliative care, with a reported prevalence of 16–55 per cent (Table 12.1).[1–5] It should be noted that oral 'discomfort' is more commonly reported than oral 'pain'.

Aetiology

Oral discomfort is often associated with xerostomia.[6] The discomfort may be related to the xerostomia per se, or to a complication of the xerostomia (e.g. oral candidosis). Oral pain can be associated with a variety of different problems. Table 12.2 shows the aetiology of oral pain in a group of patients with advanced cancer.[4]

Clinical features

Oral pain is a significant cause of morbidity in palliative care patients.[4] The morbidity relates not only to the pain, but also to the consequences of the pain: these consequences may be physical (e.g. difficulty drinking/eating), or psychological (e.g. low mood/depression).

Investigation

The assessment of oral symptoms is discussed in detail in Chapter 2. In most cases, the aetiology of the pain can be determined by the use of basic clinical skills (taking a history; performing an examination). However, occasionally, the use of investigations is required to determine the aetiology of the pain.[7]

Management

The management of oral pain involves:

- Treatment of the underlying cause
- Symptomatic treatment
  - Non-pharmacological methods – acupuncture, TENS
  - Pharmacological methods – systemic agents, topical agents

Table 12.1 Prevalence of oral discomfort/pain in palliative care patients

Study	Population type/size	Prevalence of oral discomfort/pain (%)	Comments
Gordon et al. 1985[1]	Hospice inpatients (N = 31)	55	Data refers to oral discomfort
Aldred et al. 1991[2]	Hospice inpatients (N = 20)	42	Data refers to oral soreness
Jobbins et al. 1992[3]	Hospice inpatients (N = 197)	33	Data refers to oral soreness
Oneschuk et al. 2000[4]	Advanced cancer patients (N = 99)	16	Data refers to oral pain
Davies 2000[5]	Hospital support team patients (N = 120)	46	Data refers to oral discomfort

- Anaesthetic/neurosurgical techniques – local anaesthetic blocks, neurolytic blocks.

The management of choice is treatment of the underlying cause. However, in many circumstances, there is no treatment for the underlying cause. The management of certain 'dental problems' is discussed in Chapter 4.

Painful lesions of the oral mucosa may be treated by a number of medications, both systemic and topical. An in-depth discussion of systemic analgesics is beyond the scope of this book, and readers are advised to refer to specialist palliative care/pain textbooks for further information.[7,8] Nevertheless, it is important to point out that most 'dental' pain is inflammatory in nature, and the mainstay of treatment is the use of non-steroidal anti-inflammatory drugs. Importantly, some opioid analgesics have been shown to be poorer than placebo in controlling certain types of dental pain.[9]

Topical agents may be used in isolation for mild to moderate pain (e.g. aphthous ulceration), or in combination with systemic agents for moderate to severe pain (e.g. chemotherapy-induced mucositis).[10] In the latter instance, the topical agents may have a different effect to the systemic agents, and/or may permit the dose of the systemic agents to be reduced.

Table 12.2 Aetiology of oral pain in patients with advanced cancer[4]

Aetiology of oral pain	Number of patients (N = 17)
Poorly fitting dentures	9
Oral candidosis	2
Radiation mucositis	2
Chemotherapy mucositis	1
Other (not stated)	3

The topical medications used can be classified as anaesthetic or non-anaesthetic agents. The non-anaesthetic agents include corticosteroids, non-steroidal anti-inflammatory drugs, opioids, other analgesics, and coating agents.

The choice of topical medication depends on a number of factors:[10]

◆ Disease factors – diagnosis, extent of problem

◆ Patient factors – performance status, presence of co-morbidity

◆ Drug factors – product, type of formulation.

It should be pointed out that the efficacy of a number of topical medications has not been supported by scientific evidence.

Topical local anaesthetics

Topical anaesthetics are generally applied to the oral mucosa for the following reasons: (a) to relieve the pain of oral mucosal lesions; (b) to reduce the discomfort of intra-oral local anaesthetic injections; and (c) to provide anaesthesia for operative treatment.

Both the amide and the ester classes of local anaesthetic may be used as topical anaesthetics. However, not all local anaesthetics possess a useful topical action. For example, procaine and mepivacaine cannot achieve a topical effect at clinically acceptable concentrations.[11,12]

The use of topical anaesthetics to reduce injection discomfort may not be a common practice in palliative care. Nevertheless, data from double-blind studies used to compare different topical agents to reduce injection discomfort are useful. They indicate factors that influence topical anaesthetic action. It is important to point out that such studies have investigated the efficacy of topical agents on intact mucosa. The effects on damaged, or ulcerated, mucosa may be different. The factors that influence the action of topical anaesthetics in the mouth are:

1. The drug
2. The site of application; and
3. The duration of application.

The drug

A number of studies have investigated the effects of different drugs when applied to the oral mucosa. Three aspects are relevant: (a) the anaesthetic agent used; (b) the concentration used; and (c) the formulation used.

Many studies have shown lidocaine (alone and in combination with prilocaine) and benzocaine (alone and in combination with tetracaine/amethocaine) produce anaesthesia when applied topically to oral mucosa.[13–17]

Double-blind investigations have shown an increase in efficacy when lidocaine is used in combination with prilocaine in the eutectic mixture EMLA when applied to the palate and the attached gingiva.[18,19] At the time of writing EMLA does not have a licence for intra-oral use in some countries.

Cocaine mouthwashes are sometimes used in oncology/palliative care.[20] Nevertheless, cocaine is generally not recommended for use in the mouth, because of its local vasoconstrictor, systemic stimulant, and (potentially) addictive effects.[21,22] Moreover, other local anaesthetics appear to be as effective as cocaine.

Drug concentration is important. The rate of transfer of anaesthetics applied topically is concentration-dependent.[12] There appears to be a concentration of drug above which any increase does not result in improved efficacy; up to this dose the latency of onset is decreased, and the duration of action increased, with increasing dose.[11]

Topical anaesthetics for intra-oral use can be incorporated into a number of preparations such as gels, creams, ointments, sprays, rinses, lozenges, and controlled-release devices such as impregnated patches (Fig. 12.1).[23] Different formulations vary in efficacy. For example, lower concentrations of lidocaine are needed in patches, compared to the concentration in sprays, to achieve the same level of analgesia.[24]

Controlled-release devices are designed to supply the drug at a predetermined rate over a specific time period.[25] They have been shown to be effective when applied intra-orally, and can give soft tissue anaesthesia equivalent in depth and extent to infiltration anaesthesia.[13,26]

The depth of tissue susceptible to anaesthesia produced by topical application in the mouth can be increased by the use of techniques such as iontophoresis[18,27,28]

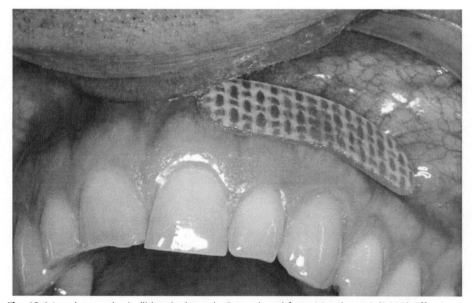

Fig. 12.1 Local anaesthetic (lidocaine) patch. Reproduced from Meechan JG (2002) Effective topical anaesthetic agents and techniques. *Dent Clin North Am* 46: 759–66, with permission.

and phonophoresis.[29] These techniques drive the agent deeper by the use of electrical current, or radio waves, respectively. Another area of development is the incorporation of topical anaesthetics into liposomes.[30–33] Progress in this field may improve the action of topical agents intra-orally.

The site of application

The effect of topical anaesthetics varies in different areas of the mouth.[11] An important factor relating to site, which influences efficacy, is the degree of keratinization of the mucosa. The palatal mucosa is much more keratinized than the buccal sulcus. Studies using lidocaine and benzocaine have shown that topical regimens that produce anaesthesia of buccal sulcus mucosa have no effect on the palate.[14,18] The degree of keratinization is not the only factor that governs efficacy. Well-designed studies have suggested the mandibular buccal sulcus is more rapidly anaesthetized following topical application compared to the equivalent zone in the maxilla.[13]

The duration of application

The depth of penetration of the applied agent is governed by the duration of application. For example, an application time of 5 minutes increases the efficacy of 5 per cent lidocaine compared to a 2 minute application.[18] Similarly, in the maxillary buccal sulcus, a 2½ minute application of a 23 mg lidocaine patch has been shown to be no better than placebo, whereas a 5 minute application achieves a pharmacological effect.[13]

One of the risks of using these agents in the oral cavity is inadvertent anaesthesia of the pharynx, which may lead to problems swallowing/aspiration of drink and food.

The systemic absorption of topical anaesthetics occurs when applied to the oral mucosa. Data from studies investigating the absorption of the anaesthetic following application to intact mucosa suggest that the anaesthetic agent does not reach therapeutic concentration in plasma in adults. Plasma concentrations are higher in children following topical application, and care must be taken not to exceed the maximum dose.[34] It is important to point out that greater levels of drug are found in the circulation after topical application to inflamed mucosa, although again in adults plasma levels approaching therapeutic concentrations are not achieved.[35]

Topical corticosteroids

Topical steroids are the mainstay of managing aphthous ulceration.[36] They appear to be most effective in treating developing lesions, rather than established lesions.[37] Topical steroids are available in a number of formulations: the potency of steroids varies from hydrocortisone (low) to clobetasol (high):[36] the preparations include creams, rinses, sprays, pellets, and adhesive tablets.[38] Topical steroids may exacerbate existing oral infections, and promote the development of oral candidosis. Hence, they should be used with caution in palliative care patients.

Topical non-steroidal anti-inflammatory drugs

Benzydamine hydrochloride

Benzydamine hydrochloride is an atypical non-steroidal anti-inflammatory drug. In addition to anti-inflammatory and analgesic properties, it possesses anaesthetic and antimicrobial properties.[39] Studies have shown it to be effective in a range of painful conditions, including aphthous ulceration,[40] chemotherapy-induced mucositis,[41] and radiation-induced mucositis.[42]

In the United Kingdom, benzydamine hydrochloride is available as a 0.15 per cent oral rinse (recommended dose: 15 ml, 1½–3 hours as required), and a 0.15 per cent spray (recommended dose: 4–8 sprays, 1½–3 hours as required).[21] The oral rinse should be maintained against the lesions for ≥ 30 sec, and then it should be expectorated (rather than swallowed).

The major side-effects of benzydamine hydrochloride are oral numbness (reported prevalence: 10 per cent), and oral burning/stinging (reported prevalence: 8 per cent).[39] Oral discomfort appears to be more of a problem in patients with extensive ulceration/inflammation. The oral discomfort can sometimes be improved by diluting the benzydamine hydrochloride with an equal volume of water.[39] It is thought that benzydamine hydrochloride does not precipitate peptic ulceration.[39]

Flurbiprofen

Flurbiprofen lozenges are indicated for the treatment of pharyngeal discomfort. The recommended dose is 1 lozenge (8.75 mg) every 3–6 hours.[21] The major side-effects of flurbiprofen are taste disturbance, and oral ulceration. It is recommended that the lozenge is moved around the mouth in order to prevent oral ulceration.[21]

Salicylates

Choline salicylate is indicated for the treatment of mild oral discomfort. It has been shown to be better than placebo in a double-blind trial involving patients with oral pain secondary to ulceration of varying causes (denture-related, traumatic, other): complete pain relief occurred in 60 per cent of the patients on active treatment, but only 9 per cent of the patients on placebo treatment.[43] The recommended dose is ½ inch (~ 1 cm) gel no more than every 3 hours.[21] The major side-effects of choline salicylate are salicylate poisoning and oral ulceration. Salicylate poisoning is associated with excessive use. Children are at greater risk of salicylate poisoning when using this product. Oral ulceration is also associated with excessive use, and with application of the gel to the mucosa beneath dentures. It is recommended that dentures be left out of the mouth for at least 30 min after application of the gel in order to prevent oral ulceration.[21]

Topical opioids

Opioids have been used topically to manage pain from a number of superficial conditions, including pain from chemotherapy-induced oral mucositis.[44] Recently, a randomized controlled trial compared a mouthwash containing morphine with a compound mouthwash in the management of chemoradiotherapy-induced oral mucositis.[45] The mouthwash containing morphine consisted of 2 per cent morphine (2 g morphine chlorhydrate diluted in 1L water), whilst the compound mouthwash consisted of a mixture of magnesium aluminium hydroxide, lidocaine and diphenhydramine. The treatment regimen consisted of holding 15 ml of the mouthwash in the mouth for 2 min every 3 hours, i.e. 6 times a day. The mouthwash containing the morphine was found to be more effective, and better tolerated, than the compound mouthwash. (The only side-effects reported with the morphine mouthwash were oral 'burning', and dry mouth).

Other topical analgesics
Capsaicin

Capsaicin is a counter irritant. It is indicated for the management of neuropathic pain (post-herpetic neuralgia, diabetic neuropathy), and has been reported as having some effect when used intraorally in the management of oral pain secondary to neuropathy[46] and chemotherapy/radiotherapy-induced mucositis.[47] Capsaicin can be used in its dermatological formulation,[46] but it has also been incorporated into an oral gel[10] and a sweet matrix.[47] One of the major (predictable) side-effects of capsaicin is an initial burning sensation. Indeed, a capsaicin-based oral pain model has been developed to assess the efficacy of other topical analgesics.[48] It is possible to overcome the initial burning sensation by the co-administration of a local anaesthetic.[10]

Doxepin

Doxepin is a tricyclic antidepressant. Its oral preparation is indicated for the management of depression, whilst its topical formulation is indicated for the management of pruritus in eczema. An oral rinse containing doxepin has been reported as having some effect when used in the management of oral pain secondary to radiation-induced mucositis and various other causes (tumour-related pain, chemotherapy-related mucositis, graft-versus-host disease).[49] The reported side-effects of topical doxepin include oral discomfort, taste disturbance and sedation.[49]

Coating agents

Coating agents primarily act by forming a barrier over oral ulcers, thereby protecting them from trauma and other irritants. If trauma and other irritants are a major cause of discomfort, then such agents may be effective (e.g. aphthous ulceration). However, the effectiveness of such agents is dependent on their ability to bind/remain bound to the ulcerated lesions. If the underlying disease process is the major cause of discomfort, then such agents will be relatively ineffective (e.g. chemotherapy-induced mucositis).

Carbenoxolone

Carbenoxolone has been shown to have some effect in aphthous ulceration[50] and also in oral herpes simplex infection.[51] It is thought that the improvement in oral discomfort is due to a combination of the coating effect of the drug, and also the disease-modifying effects of the drug. For example, carbenoxolone appears to have an antiviral action, which may help to explain its efficacy in oral herpes simplex infection.[51] Carbenoxolone is available as a gel for localized problems, and a mouthwash for more widespread problems. The gel/mouthwash are applied after meals, and at bedtime.

Carmellose sodium

Carmellose sodium (with gelatin and pectin) is available for topical use in the mouth in the form of a paste, and also a powder. It is recommended that a thin layer of the paste is applied to, or the powder sprinkled on, the painful areas after meals.[21]

Sucralfate

Sucralfate has been shown to have some effect in aphthous ulceration.[52] However, studies suggest that sucralfate has little effect in chemotherapy-induced mucositis[53] and also in radiation-induced mucositis.[54] Indeed, its use in these circumstances has been discouraged.[55]

Gelclair®

Gelclair® is a relatively new product, which contains both polvinylpyrrolidone and sodium hyaluronate. It has been reported to reduce pain from a variety of different oral pathologies.[56] Currently, this product is the subject of randomized controlled trials in the management of chemotherapy-induced mucositis, and radiation-induced mucositis.

Other topical agents

Other recommended options for treating oral discomfort include rinsing the mouth with warm normal saline, or warm dilute compound thymol glycerin.[21]

Diphenhydramine (an antihistamine) is often included in preparations used to treat cancer treatment-related mucositis.[45,57]

Local anaesthetic blocks

The use of local anaesthetic techniques should be considered as a temporary measure for control of oral pain until definitive measures can be performed. Conventional agents such as lidocaine with epinephrine will produce soft tissue anaesthesia of 2–3 hours, and good bony and dental anaesthesia of around 45 minutes. The so-called 'long-acting' agents, such as bupivacaine, can produce anaesthesia of around 6 hours.

An in-depth discussion of relevant local anaesthetic blocks is beyond the scope of this book, and readers are advised to refer to a specialist dental textbook for further information.[22]

Neurolytic blocks

The use of neurolytic agents is uncommon in the control of oral pain, although they have been shown to be effective in the management of trigeminal neuralgia[7] and pain due to local tumour.[58] Again, an in-depth discussion of relevant neurolytic blocks is beyond the scope of this book, and readers are advised to refer to a specialist pain textbook for further information.[7,58]

References

1. Gordon SR, Berkey DB, Call RL (1985). Dental need among hospice patients in Colorado: a pilot study. *Gerodontics* **1**: 125–9.

2. Aldred MJ, Addy M, Bagg J, Finlay I (1991). Oral health in the terminally ill: a cross-sectional pilot survey. *Spec Care Dentist* **11**: 59–62.

3. Jobbins J, Bagg J, Finlay IG, Addy M, Newcombe RG (1992). Oral and dental disease in terminally ill cancer patients. *BMJ* **304**: 1612.

4. Oneschuk D, Hanson J, Bruera E (2000). A survey of mouth pain and dryness in patients with advanced cancer. *Support Care Cancer* **8**: 372–6.

5. Davies ANT (2000). An investigation into the relationship between salivary gland hypofunction and oral health problems in patients with advanced cancer. Dissertation. King's College: University of London.

6. Davies AN, Broadley K, Beighton D (2001). Xerostomia in patients with advanced cancer. *J Pain Symptom Manage* **22**: 820–5.

7. Zakrzewska JM, Harrison SD (2002). *Assessment and Management of Orofacial Pain*. Amsterdam: Elsevier Science B.V.

8. Doyle D, Hanks G, Cherny N, Calman K (2003). *Oxford Textbook of Palliative Medicine*, 3rd edn. Oxford: Oxford University Press.

9. Seymour RA, Rawlins MD, Rowell FJ (1982). Dihydrocodeine-induced hyperalgesia in post-operative dental pain. *Lancet* **1**: 1425–6.

10. Padilla M, Clark GT, Merrill RL (2000). Topical medications for orofacial neuropathic pain: a review. *J Am Dent Assoc* **131**: 184–95.

11. Bergman S, Kane D, Siegal IA, Ciancio S (1969). In vitro and in situ transfer of local anaesthetics across the oral mucosa. *Arch Oral Biol* **14**: 35–43.

12. Bjerring P, Arendt-Nielsen L (1990). Depth and duration of skin analgesia to needle insertion after topical application of EMLA cream. *Br J Anaesth* **64**: 173–7.

13. Hersh EV, Houpt MI, Cooper SA, Feldman RS, Wolff MS, Levin LM (1996). Analgesic efficacy and safety of an intraoral lidocaine patch. *J Am Dent Assoc* **127**: 1626–34.

14. Hutchins HS Jr, Young FA, Lackland DT, Fishburne CP (1997). The effectiveness of topical anesthesia and vibration in alleviating the pain of oral injections. *Anesth Prog* **44**: 87–9.

15. Rosivack RG, Koenigsberg SR, Maxwell KC (1990). An analysis of the effectiveness of two topical anesthetics. *Anesth Prog* **37**: 290–2.

16. Svensson P, Petersen JK (1992). Anesthetic effect of EMLA occluded with Orahesive oral bandages on oral mucosa. A placebo-controlled study. *Anesth Prog* **39**: 79–82.

17. Vickers ER, Punnia-Moorthy A (1992). A clinical evaluation of three topical anaesthetic agents. *Aust Dent J* **37**: 267–70.

18. Holst A, Evers H (1985). Experimental studies of new topical anaesthetics on the oral mucosa. *Swed Dent J* **9**: 185–91.

19. Meechan JG, Thomason JM (1999). A comparison of two topical anesthetics on the discomfort of intraligamentary injections: a double-blind split-mouth volunteer clinical trial. *Oral Surg Oral Med Oral Pathol Oral Radiol Endod* **87**: 362–5.

20. Twycross R, Wilcock A, Charlesworth S, Dickman A (2002). *Palliative Care Formulary*, 2nd edn. Oxford: Radcliffe Medical Press.

21. Anonymous (2003). *British National Formulary* 46 (September 2003). London: British Medical Association and the Royal Pharmaceutical Society of Great Britain.

22. Meechan JG, Robb ND, Seymour RA (1998). *Pain and Anxiety Control for the Conscious Dental Patient*. Oxford: Oxford University Press.

23. Meechan JG (2002). Effective topical anesthetic agents and techniques. *Dent Clin North Am* **46**: 759–66.

24. Giddon DB, Quadland M, Rachwall PC, Springer J, Tursky B (1968). Development of a method for comparing topical anesthetics in different application and dosage forms. *J Oral Ther Pharmacol* **4**: 270–4.

25. Brook IM, van Noort R (1984). Controlled delivery of drugs. A review of polymer-based devices. *Br Dent J* **157**: 11–15.

26. Brook IM, Tucker GT, Tuckley EC, Boyes RN (1989). A lignocaine patch for dental analgesia safety and early pharmacology. *J Control Release* **10**: 183–8.

27. Kincheloe JE, Mealiea WL Jr, Mattison GD, Seib K (1991). Psychophysical measurement on pain perception after administration of a topical anesthetic. *Quintessence Int* **22**: 311–15.

28. Won SH, Ryu HR, Lee SW, Kho HS (1995). Penetration of lidocaine into oral mucosa by iontophoresis and its clinical application. *J Dent Res* **74**: 576.

29. Malamed SF (1992). What's new in local anesthesia? *Anesth Prog* **39**: 125–31.

30. Lener EV, Bucalo BD, Kist DA, Moy RL (1997). Topical anesthetic agents in dermatologic surgery. A review. *Dermatol Surg* **23**: 673–83.

31. Gesztes A, Mezei M (1988). Topical anesthesia of the skin by liposome-encapsulated tetracaine. *Anesth Analg* **67**: 1079–81.

32. Hung OR, Comeau L, Riley MR, Tan S, Whynot S, Mezei M (1997). Comparative topical anaesthesia of EMLA and liposome-encapsulated tetracaine. *Can J Anaesth* **44**: 707–11.

33. Zed CM, Epstein J, Donaldson D (1996). Topical liposome encapsulated tetracaine versus benzocaine – a clinical investigation. *J Dent Res* **75**: 247.

34. Leopold A, Wilson S, Weaver JS, Moursi AM (2002). Pharmacokinetics of lidocaine delivered from a transmucosal patch in children. *Anesth Prog* **49**: 82–7.

35. Elad S, Cohen G, Zylber-Katz E, Findler M, Galili D, Garfunkel AA *et al.* (1999). Systemic absorption of lidocaine after topical application for the treatment of oral mucositis in bone marrow transplantation patients. *J Oral Pathol Med* **28**: 170–2.

36. Ship JA (1996). Recurrent aphthous stomatitis. An update. *Oral Surg Oral Med Oral Pathol Oral Radiol Endod* **82**: 141–7.

37. Holbrook WP, Kristmundsdottir T, Loftsson T (1998). Aqueous hydrocortisone mouthwash solution: clinical evaluation. *Acta Odontol Scand* **56**: 157–60.

38. Ceschel GC, Maffei P, Lombardi Biogia S, Ronchi C (2001). Design and evaluation of buccal adhesive hydrocortisone acetate (HCA) tablets. *Drug Deliv* **8**: 161–71.

39. Turnball RS (1995). Benzydamine hydrochloride (Tantum) in the management of oral inflammatory conditions. *J Can Dent Assoc* **61**: 127–34.

40. Yankell SL, Welsh CA, Cohen DW (1981). Evaluation of benzydamine HCl in patients with aphthous ulcers. *Compend Contin Educ Dent* **2**: 14–16.

41. Sonis ST, Clairmont F, Lockhart PB, Connolly SF (1985). Benzydamine HCl in the management of chemotherapy-induced mucositis. *J Oral Med* **40**: 67–71.

42. Kim JH, Chu F, Lakshmi V, Houde R (1985). A clinical study of benzydamine for the treatment of radiotherapy-induced mucositis of the oropharynx. *Int J Tissue React* **7**: 215–18.

43. Jolley HM, Torneck CD, Siegel I (1972). A topical choline salicylate gel for control of pain and inflammation in oral conditions – a controlled study. *J Can Dent Assoc* **38**: 72–4.

44. Krajnik M, Zylicz Z, Finlay I, Luczak J, van Sorge AA (1999). Potential uses of topical opioids in palliative care – report of six cases. *Pain* **80**: 121–5.

45. Cerchietti LC, Navigante AH, Bonomi MR, Zaderajko MA, Menendez PR, Pogany CE *et al.* (2002). Effect of topical morphine for mucositis-associated pain following concomitant chemoradiotherapy for head and neck carcinoma. *Cancer* **95**: 2230–6.

46. Epstein JB, Marcoe JH (1994). Topical application of capsaicin for treatment of oral neuropathic pain and trigeminal neuralgia. *Oral Surg Oral Med Oral Pathol* **77**: 135–40.

47. Berger A, Henderson M, Nadoolman W, Duffy V, Cooper D, Saberski L *et al.* (1995). Oral capsaicin provides temporary relief for oral mucositis pain secondary to chemotherapy/radiation therapy. *J Pain Symptom Manage* **10**: 243–8.

48. Ngom PI, Dubray C, Woda A, Dallel R (2001). A human oral capsaicin pain model to assess topical anesthetic-analgesic drugs. *Neurosci Lett* **316**: 149–52.

49. Epstein JB, Truelove EL, Oien H, Allison C, Le ND, Epstein MS (2001). Oral topical doxepin rinse: analgesic effect in patients with oral mucosal pain due to cancer or cancer therapy. *Oral Oncol* **37**: 632–7.

50. Poswillo D, Partridge M (1984). Management of recurrent aphthous ulcers. A trial of carbenoxolone sodium mouthwash. *Br Dent J* **157**: 55–7.

51. Partridge M, Poswillo DE (1984). Topical carbenoxolone sodium in the management of herpes simplex infection. *Br J Oral Maxillofac Surg* **22**: 138–45.

52. Rattan J, Schneider M, Arber N, Gorsky M, Dayan D (1994). Sucralfate suspension as a treatment of recurrent aphthous stomatitis. *J Intern Med* **236**: 341–3.

53. Loprinzi CL, Ghosh C, Camoriano J, Sloan J, Steen PD, Michalak JC *et al.* (1997). Phase III controlled evaluation of sucralfate to alleviate stomatitis in patients receiving fluorouracil-based chemotherapy. *J Clin Oncol* **15**: 1235–8.

54. Franzen L, Henriksson R, Littbrand B, Zackrisson B (1995). Effects of sucralfate on mucositis during and following radiotherapy of malignancies in the head and neck region. *Acta Oncol* **34**: 219–23.

55. Rubenstein EB (1998). Evaluating cost-effectiveness in outpatient management of medical complications in cancer patients. *Curr Opin Oncol* **10**: 297–301.

56. Innocenti M, Moscatelli G, Lopez S (2002). Efficacy of Gelclair in reducing pain in palliative care patients with oral lesions: preliminary findings from an open pilot study. *J Pain Symptom Manage* **24**: 456–7.

57. Dodd MJ, Dibble SL, Miaskowski C, MacPhail L, Greenspan D, Paul SM *et al.* (2000). Randomized clinical trial of the effectiveness of three commonly used mouthwashes to treat chemotherapy-induced mucositis. *Oral Surg Oral Med Oral Pathol Oral Radiol Endod* **90**: 39–47.

58. Wall PD, Melzack R (1999). *Textbook of Pain*, 4th edn. Edinburgh: Churchill Livingstone.

Useful websites

British National Formulary
http://www.bnf.org

Chapter 13

Miscellaneous oral problems

Anita Sengupta and John Eveson

Burning mouth syndrome[1]

- *Synonyms* – burning mouth, burning tongue, sore tongue, glossodynia, oral dysaesthesia, stomatodynia, glossopyrosis.

- *Definition* – Burning mouth syndrome is 'an intra-oral burning sensation for which no medical or odontological causes can be found and in which the oral mucosa is of grossly normal appearance'.

- *Epidemiology* – Burning mouth is a common symptom (~15 per cent population). However, burning mouth syndrome is a less common problem (~1 per cent population). It is associated with female gender and increasing age.

- *Aetiology* – The cause is unknown. Various local factors have been implicated, including nerve damage and xerostomia. Similarly, various systemic factors have been implicated, including psychological problems and the menopause.

- *Clinical features* – The characteristic features of burning mouth syndrome are shown in Table 13.1. Patients may also complain of oral paraesthesia, xerostomia, dysgeusia, or dysosmia (altered smell).

- *Investigation* – It is essential to differentiate between burning mouth and burning mouth syndrome. The assessment of burning mouth involves taking a history, performing an examination, and the use of appropriate investigations (see Chapter 2). Routine investigations include a full blood count, serum ferritin, red cell folate, and serum vitamin B12. Other investigations are dependent on the findings from the history and examination.

- *Management* – A variety of different modalities have been used to treat burning mouth syndrome. There is some evidence to support the use of cognitive behavioural therapy, but less evidence to support the use of analgesics/adjuvant analgesics. Drugs that are often employed include antidepressants (e.g. amitriptyline), and anticonvulsants (e.g. clonazepam). About 1/3 –1/2 of patients improve over time, although it may take several years for the improvement to occur.

Table 13.1 Clinical features of burning mouth syndrome[1]

Clinical features		
History	Onset	Gradual (months to years)
	Temporal pattern	Intermittent/continuous
		Often worse in evening
	Site	Tongue/other sites
		Often multifocal
	Radiation	Intra-oral
	Quality/character	Burning, smarting, tender, annoying
	Intensity/severity	Mild/moderate
	Aggravating factors	Stress, fatigue
	Relieving factors	Sleep, distraction, cold drink/food
Examination	Oral examination	Normal

Racial pigmentation[2]

◆ *Epidemiology* – Common. Occurs in people of African, Asian, and Southern European descent.

◆ *Clinical features* – Asymptomatic. The most common site is the gingivae (Fig. 13.1). Other common sites are the buccal mucosa and the palatal mucosa; less common sites are the lips, the tongue, and the floor of mouth. The areas of

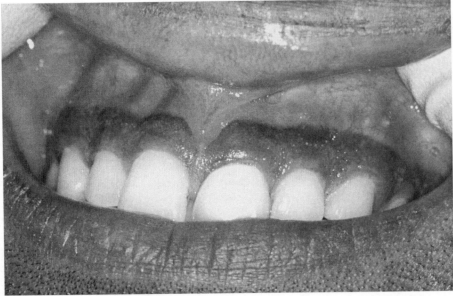

Fig. 13.1 Racial pigmentation. Courtesy of J Eveson. (See also Plate 25 at the centre of this book.)

pigmentation are variable in size, but are usually symmetrical in distribution. Over time, the lesions may darken in colour.

+ *Management* – No treatment is required (reassurance).

Oral varicosities[3]

+ *Synonyms* – Varices, venous lakes.

+ *Epidemiology* – Common. Occurs in older people (>50 yr).

+ *Aetiology* – The lesions are due to dilatation of superficial veins.

+ *Clinical features* – Asymptomatic. The most common sites are the lips and the ventral surface of the tongue. However, they can occur elsewhere within the oral cavity. On the lips they appear as blue/purple swellings, which blanch on pressure (Fig. 13.2); on the tongue they appear as dilated, tortuous veins. Over time, the lesions may become more conspicuous. Oral varicosities occasionally thrombose, but rarely haemorrhage.

+ *Management* – Usually, no treatment is required (reassurance). Sometimes, treatment is given for aesthetic reasons for lesions on the lips, i.e. excision, cryotherapy, or laser therapy.

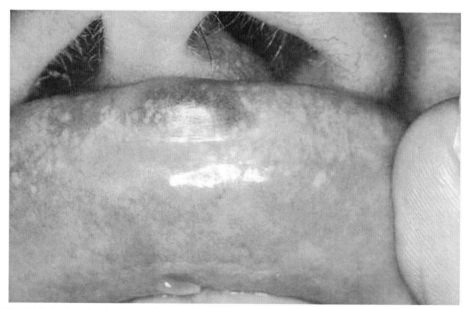

Fig. 13.2 Oral varicosity. Reproduced with permission from MP Sweeney and J Bagg (1997) *Making Sense of the Mouth*, Partnership in Oral Care, Glasgow. (See also Plate 26 at the centre of this book.)

Recurrent aphthous ulcers[4]

- *Synonyms* – Recurrent aphthous stomatitis, recurrent oral ulceration.
- *Epidemiology* – Very common (10–30 per cent population). More common in young adults and in females.
- *Aetiology* – The cause is unknown. (Some patients have iron, folate or vitamin B12 deficiency). Attacks may be precipitated by stress, trauma, and menstruation.
- *Clinical features* – Recurrent aphthous ulcers have been classified into three main types: (1) minor; (2) major; and (3) herpetiform. The clinical features of the different types of recurrent aphthous ulcers are shown in Table 13.2. (Fig. 13.3).
- *Management* – Various agents have been used to treat aphthous ulceration. Topical corticosteroids are the mainstay of treatment, whilst systemic corticosteroids are reserved for treatment of severe/refractory cases. Other agents that have been used include topical analgesics, systemic analgesics, tetracycline mouthwashes, and thalidomide (see Chapter 12).

Neutropenic ulcers[5]

- *Epidemiology* – Common (in high risk groups).
- *Aetiology* – The lesions are related to low neutrophil counts. However, in ~ one-third of cases, additional factors appear to be relevant (e.g. trauma, infection). The underlying causes of the neutropenia, include inherited disorders (e.g. cyclic neutropenia), and acquired disorders (e.g. bone marrow infiltration with cancer, bone marrow suppression with cancer chemotherapy).
- *Clinical features* – Neutropenic ulcers are often painful, and may be associated with other oral symptoms (hypersalivation, difficulty eating). The ulcers vary in number (often multiple), in size (often large), and in site: the most common sites are the gingivae, the tongue, the palate and the tonsils. The edge of the ulcer is usually well demarcated, although there are few signs of surrounding inflammation. The base of the ulcer is usually covered with a grey-white/yellow pseudomembrane. Neutropenic ulcers are often associated with other relevant oral pathology (gingivitis, mucositis).
- *Management* – The management of neutropenic ulcers is essentially symptomatic (good oral hygiene, topical corticosteroids, topical analgesics). Improvement in the neutrophil count is associated with improvement in the neutropenic ulcers. Granulocyte-colony stimulating factors may be useful in treating neutropenia secondary to bone marrow suppression with cancer chemotherapy.

Table 13.2 Clinical features of recurrent aphthous ulcers[10]

Type	Site	Number	Size	Characteristics	Natural history	Other comments
Minor	Lip, buccal mucosa, tongue, mucolabial fold, mucobuccal fold	1–6	Medium (2–6mm)	Oval Narrow red margin Shallow base White-yellow pseudomembrane	Persist 5–7 days Often recur every few months	Most common type A burning sensation may precede (24–48hr) the ulceration Very painful
Major	Lip, buccal mucosa, tongue, soft palate	1–5	Large (1–2cm)	Deep base Ulcers may heal by scarring	Persist 3–6 weeks Often recur every few months	Very painful
Herpetiform	Anywhere in oral cavity	10–100	Small (1–2mm)	Shallow base Ulcers may coalesce to form larger lesions	Persist 1–2 weeks Attacks recur over period of 1–3 yr	Very painful

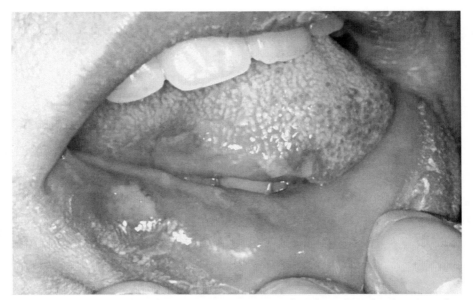

Fig. 13.3 Recurrent minor aphthous ulceration. Courtesy of J Eveson. (See also Plate 27 at the centre of this book.)

Fissured tongue[6]

- *Synonym* – Scrotal tongue.
- *Epidemiology* – Relatively common (0.5–5 per cent population). Associated with Down's syndrome, and Melkersson–Rosenthal syndrome.
- *Aetiology* – Developmental anomaly. The cause is unknown. May be familial.
- *Clinical features* – Generally asymptomatic, although patients sometimes complain of discomfort. There are multiple fissures on dorsal surface of tongue (Fig. 13.4). The fissures are variable in number, size and depth, but are usually symmetrical in distribution. Fissured tongue may coexist with geographic tongue.
- *Management* – None required (reassurance).

Geographical tongue[7]

- *Synonyms* – Benign migratory glossitis, erythema migrans.
- *Epidemiology* – Relatively common (1–2 per cent population). Associated with psoriasis.

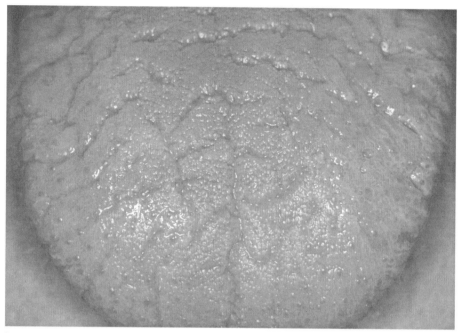

Fig. 13.4 Fissured tongue. Courtesy of J Eveson. (See also Plate 28 at the centre of this book.)

- *Aetiology* – The lesions are due to desquamation of the filiform papillae. The cause is unknown. May be familial.
- *Clinical features* – Generally asymptomatic, although patients sometimes complain of discomfort. There are multiple, irregularly shaped, patches on the dorsal surface of the tongue: the patches have a narrow, raised, white edge, and a smooth, flat, erythematous centre (Fig. 13.5). Geographic tongue is a dynamic condition: patches appear then disappear; patches change size and/or shape. Similar lesions may occur on the lateral/ventral surface of tongue, and on the remaining oral mucosa ('geographic stomatitis'). Geographic tongue is often intermittent, and often resolves spontaneously (weeks to years). Geographic tongue may coexist with fissured tongue.
- *Management* – None required (reassurance).

Black hairy tongue[8]

- *Synonyms* – Hairy tongue, brown hairy tongue.
- *Epidemiology* – Relatively common.

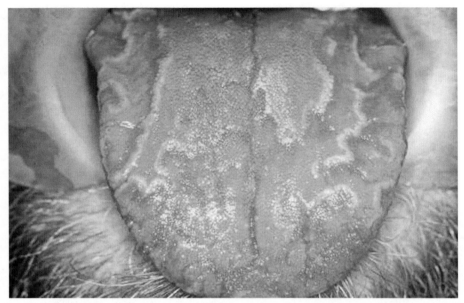

Fig. 13.5 Geographic tongue. Reproduced with permission from MP Sweeney and J Bagg (1997) *Making Sense of the Mouth*, Partnership in Oral Care, Glasgow. (See also Plate 29 at the centre of this book.)

- *Aetiology* – The lesions are due to hypertrophy/elongation of the filiform papillae. The discolouration may be due to overgrowth of chromogenic bacteria, or to pigments derived from eating/smoking. The cause unknown, although it is associated with smoking, antibiotic use, other drug use (e.g. ferrous sulphate), and poor oral hygiene.
- *Clinical features* – Generally asymptomatic, although some patients complain of discomfort/taste disturbance. There is a 'hairy' patch in the central, posterior part of the dorsal surface of the tongue. The 'hairs' are yellow, brown, or black in colour (Fig. 13.6).
- *Management* – Treatment involves oral hygiene measures, including tongue cleaning (brushing, scraping). Associated factors should be discontinued/avoided.

Stomatitis nicotina[9]

- *Synonyms* – Nicotinic stomatitis, smoker's palate, smoker's keratosis, stomatitis palatini.
- *Epidemiology* – Uncommon. Mainly occurs in pipe smokers, although it can occur in cigar/cigarette smokers.

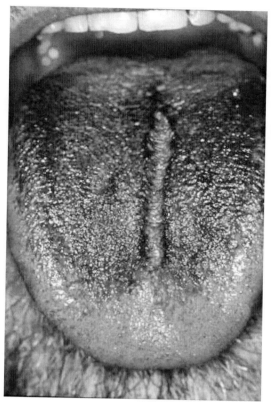

Fig. 13.6 Black hairy tongue. Reproduced with permission from MP Sweeney and J Bagg (1997) *Making Sense of the Mouth*, Partnership in Oral Care, Glasgow. (See also Plate 30 at the centre of this book.)

- *Aetiology* – The lesion is due primarily to keratosis of the mucosa, and secondarily to inflammation of the minor salivary glands. It is thought that the underlying cause is the heat generated by the pipe, although there may be a contribution from the chemicals generated by the tobacco.

- *Clinical features* – Asymptomatic. The lesion involves the palate. The keratosis results in a white, multi-nodular, fissured appearance of the mucosa, whilst the inflammation of the minor salivary glands results in red 'spots' within the mucosa (Fig. 13.7). Stomatitis nicotina is not a pre-malignant condition, although it may be associated with other smoking-related, pre-malignant conditions (oral leukoplakia).

- *Management* – Cessation of smoking. (Cessation of smoking leads to rapid regression of the lesion).

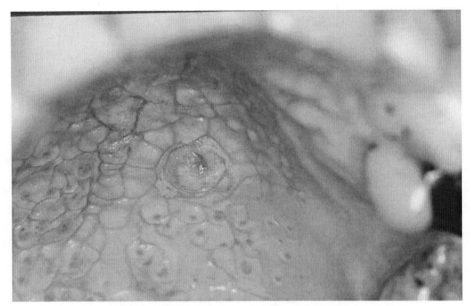

Fig. 13.7 Stomatitis nicotina. Reproduced with permission from MP Sweeney and J Bagg (1997) *Making Sense of the Mouth*, Partnership in Oral Care, Glasgow. (See also Plate 31 at the centre of this book.)

References

1. Zakrzewska JM (2002). Burning mouth. In JM Zakrzewska, SD Harrison (ed.) *Assessment and Management of Orofacial Pain*. Amsterdam: Elsevier Science BV.

2. Amir E, Gorsky M, Buchner A, Sarnat H, Gat H (1991). Physiologic pigmentation of the oral mucosa in Israeli children. *Oral Surg Oral Med Oral Pathol* **71**: 396–8.

3. del Pozo J, Pena C, Garcia Silva J, Goday JJ, Fonseca E (2003). Venous lakes: a report of 32 cases treated by carbon dioxide laser vaporization. *Dermatol Surg* **29**: 308–10.

4. Ship JA, Chavez EM, Doerr PA, Henson BS, Sarmadi M (2000). Recurrent aphthous stomatitis. *Quintessence Int* **31**: 95–112.

5. DeConno F, Sbanotto A, Ripamonti C, Ventafridda V (2003). Mouth care. In D Doyle, G Hanks, N Cherny, K Calman (ed.) *Oxford Textbook of Palliative Medicine*, 3rd edn. Oxford: Oxford University Press.

6. Leston JM, Santos AA, Varela-Centelles PI, Garcia JV, Romero MA, Villamor LP (2002). Oral mucosa: variations from normalcy, part II. *Cutis* **69**: 215–17.

7. Assimakopoulos D, Patrikakos G, Fotika C, Elisaf M (2002). Benign migratory glossitis or geographic tongue: an enigmatic oral lesion. *Am J Med* **113**: 751–5.

8. Sarti GM, Haddy RI, Schaffer D, Kihm J (1990). Black hairy tongue. *Am Fam Physician* **41**: 1751–5.

9. Taybos G (2003). Oral changes associated with tobacco use. *Am J Med Sci* **326**: 179–82.
10. Laskaris G (1994). *Colour Atlas of Oral Diseases*, 2nd edn. Stuttgart: Georg Thieme Verlag.

Useful websites

European Association of Oral Medicine
http://www.eastman.ucl.ac.uk/~eaom

Chapter 14

Head and neck cancer

Jan Roodenburg and Andrew Davies

Introduction

The term 'head and neck cancer' has been variously used to describe all malignant tumours within the region, or merely malignant tumours arising from the upper aerodigestive tract. The focus of this chapter will be on patients with carcinomas arising from the upper aerodigestive tract, since this is the group of patients that are most often referred for specialist palliative care.

Head and neck cancers are relatively uncommon in many parts of the developed world. For example, they account for <5 per cent of malignant tumours in the United Kingdom.[1] Nevertheless, head and neck cancers present particular challenges to healthcare professionals as a result of various disease-related factors (tumour site, tumour biology), treatment-related factors (morbidity), and patient-related factors (co-morbidity).

Patients often present with locally advanced disease, but rarely with distant metastatic disease. Nevertheless, the prognosis is relatively poor in this group of patients (overall five year survival ~ 40 per cent).[2] The poor prognosis is related both to progression of the malignant disease, and also to development/progression of associated diseases (e.g. lung cancer, ischaemic heart disease, chronic obstructive pulmonary disease).[1]

The first part of the chapter will discuss the principles of management of head and neck cancer, whilst the second part of the chapter will discuss the palliative care of patients with advanced head and neck cancer.

Generic issues
Strategy of treatment

The initial management of patients with head and neck cancer depends on a number of factors, including tumour histology, tumour site, tumour stage, and presence of co-morbidity. The options for treatment include surgery, radiotherapy, chemotherapy, other anticancer therapies, or a combination of these interventions. The reader is advised to refer to a specialist textbook for detailed information about the management of head and neck cancer.[3,4]

The decision about embarking on a course of treatment is relatively straightforward for patients with early disease, where the aim of treatment is cure, and the pros of treatment generally outweigh the cons of treatment (i.e. inconvenience, morbidity, mortality). However, it is much less straightforward for patients with late/recurrent disease, where the aim of treatment is palliation. Thus, treatment given with a palliative intent can be radical in nature, i.e. major surgery, prolonged course of radiotherapy.

It is important that all of the options are debated within the multidisciplinary team (see below), and that all of the options are presented to the patient and their family. Moreover, it is important that patients are given an honest appraisal of the efficacy/morbidity of each option.

Surgery

Surgery is mainly employed as primary treatment for loco-regional disease. It is often supplemented with postoperative radiotherapy in locally advanced disease. Surgery may also be used to treat persistent disease following radiotherapy ('salvage surgery'), to treat recurrent disease, and to manage specific problems, e.g. fistula, haemorrhage.

Modern head and neck cancer surgery is based on the '3 R's' principles: (1) Resection; (2) Reconstruction; and (3) Rehabilitation. Thus, the aims of treatment are to completely resect the tumour, to reconstruct the defect so that the patient's appearance/function is as good as possible, and to rehabilitate the patient so that they can lead as normal a life as possible. Numerous studies have demonstrated the importance of the type of resection, the method of reconstruction, and the type of rehabilitation on subsequent quality of life. A variety of different techniques are involved in rehabilitation, including the provision of intra-oral prosthesis to aid oral function, and facial prostheses to aid cosmesis.[5]

Head and neck surgery is associated with a wide range of clinically important side-effects (acute and chronic).[6] In particular, head and neck surgery may result in ongoing facial disfigurement, and functional impairment (see below). Surgery in patients with advanced disease is associated with an increased incidence of complications, as a result of the poor condition of the patients. Similarly 'salvage surgery' is associated with an increased incidence of complications, as a result of impaired blood supply and healing mechanisms (i.e. delayed healing, wound breakdown, and fistula formation).

Radiotherapy

Radiotherapy is employed as primary treatment for loco-regional disease, particularly where surgery is impracticable, or where surgery would result in unacceptable cosmesis and/or functional impairment.[7] It is often used to supplement surgery in locally advanced disease. Radiotherapy may also be used to treat recurrent disease and to manage specific problems, e.g. pain, haemorrhage.

A variety of different techniques (external beam, brachytherapy), fractionation schedules (conventional, hyperfraction) and concomitant therapies (transfusion, chemotherapy) have been employed to try to improve the outcomes of radiotherapy.[7] Most patients are treated with a radical (prolonged) course of radiotherapy, although some patients with advanced disease/poor prognosis are treated with a palliative (short) course of radiotherapy. It should be noted that palliative courses of radiotherapy do not provide long-term palliation of symptoms, because of rapid regrowth of the tumour.

Head and neck radiotherapy is associated with a wide range of clinically important side-effects (acute and chronic).[7] Radiation-induced side-effects are discussed in detail in Chapter 15. Concomitant treatment with chemotherapy is associated with an increased incidence of complications. Similarly, re-irradiation is associated with an increased incidence of complications, as a result of normal tissue tolerances.

Chemotherapy

The role of chemotherapy in the management of head and neck cancer remains to be determined.[8] Currently, chemotherapy is employed in radical regimens aimed at curing the disease, and also in palliative regimens aimed at symptom control.

Delivery of treatment

Multidisciplinary teams

The appropriate management of head and neck cancer relies on the input of a wide range of professionals. The core multidisciplinary team includes ENT surgeons, oromaxillofacial surgeons, plastic surgeons, clinical oncologists, clinical nurse specialists, dentists, dieticians, speech and language therapists, palliative care specialists, radiologists and pathologists. However, other professionals may be required from time to time, e.g. prosthetic specialists.

It is important that all new patients are assessed/discussed by the whole multidisciplinary team. Moreover, it is equally important that patients have access to these professionals throughout their illness, particularly during the terminal phase of the disease. The multidisciplinary team must liase with the primary care team, in order to ensure continuity of care for these patients.

Specialist centres

Increasingly, there has been a move towards treating patients with head and neck cancer in specialist centres, rather than in local units. The rationale for this change includes the small number of cases, and the necessary infrastructure for providing appropriate care for such patients (multidisciplinary teams, specialist facilities). Evidence is now emerging that specialist units produce better results than local units (Prof. Martin Birchall, personal communication).

Whilst it may be appropriate for patients with early (curable) disease to be treated at a specialist centre some distance from their home, it would more appropriate for patients with advanced (incurable) disease to be treated at the local unit. Thus, it is important that there is good communication between the specialist unit and the local units, and that relevant professionals/services remain accessible at the local units.

Specific problems

Patients with advanced head and neck cancer may experience a number of physical, psychological, social and spiritual problems. The physical problems may be due to an effect of the cancer (direct, indirect), an effect of the cancer treatment, an effect of a concomitant disorder, or a combination of the aforementioned factors.

Pain

Pain is the most common symptom in patients with advanced head and neck cancer. Thus, studies have reported prevalences of 79–85 per cent.[9,10]

Patients often experience multiple pains, of varying causes, and of varying types. Grond et al. reported that the main cause of pain in their patients was a direct effect of the cancer (72 per cent).[11] Other causes of pain included an indirect effect of the cancer (2 per cent), the cancer treatment (19 per cent), and a concomitant disease (4 per cent). Grond et al. also reported that the main type of pain in their patients was nociceptive in nature (75 per cent).[11]

The management of pain involves treatment of the underlying cause, and/or symptomatic treatment. In most cases, the pain responds to conventional analgesic regimens (e.g. WHO guidelines).[11,12] Nevertheless, in some cases, the pain requires more interventional approaches (e.g. neurolytic procedures).[13,14] The management of oral pain is discussed in detail in Chapter 12.

Airway problems

Airway obstruction is a common problem in head and neck cancer patients. Thus, Aird et al. reported an incidence of 28 per cent amongst their cohort of patients.[15] However, airway obstruction is a relatively uncommon cause of death in head and neck cancer patients (see below).[9]

The management of airway obstruction includes treatment of the underlying cancer, performance of a tracheostomy, and/or symptomatic management. It is important that a management plan is developed for patients at risk of airway obstruction. It is equally important that the management plan is reassessed on a regular basis.

Ideally, a tracheostomy should be performed before the airway becomes dangerously compromised. A fenestrated tracheostomy tube should be used, so that the patient can continue to communicate verbally (Fig. 14.1). Ongoing care of the tracheostomy/airways should help to diminish further problems, e.g. cleaning of the tube, humidification of the air, physiotherapy, suction.[16]

In cases of subacute obstruction, where performance of a tracheostomy is not indicated, various interventions may be used to try to alleviate the patient's distress, e.g. corticosteroids, helium and oxygen mixtures.[17] In addition, interventions used to treat dyspnoea may be of benefit in this situation, e.g. opioids, benzodiazepines.[18]

In cases of acute obstruction, where performance of a tracheostomy is not indicated, and where the patient is in extremis, a sedative drug should be used to alleviate the

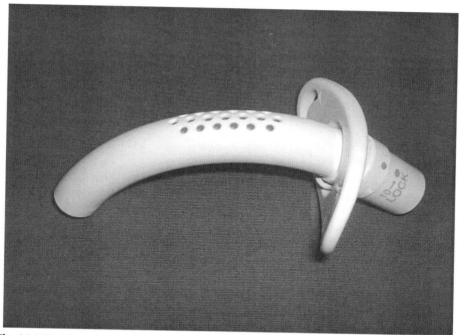

Fig. 14.1 Fenestrated tracheostomy tube.

patient's distress, e.g. midazolam.[19] In most cases, a subcutaneous injection of 2.5–5 mg of midazolam will adequately sedate the patient. However, some patients require further/larger doses of midazolam, e.g. patients on long-term benzodiazepine therapy.

It should be noted that head and neck patients may have other causes for respiratory distress including chronic obstructive pulmonary disease, lung cancer, pulmonary embolus, and aspiration pneumonia (secondary to dysphagia).

Nutritional problems

Nutritional problems are very common in patients with advanced head and neck cancer.[9,10]

Dysphagia is the major cause of nutritional problems in this group of patients. For example, Forbes reported a prevalence of 74 per cent amongst a cohort of patients with advanced disease.[9] Dysphagia is generally related to damage to oropharyngeal structures, damage to nerve supply of oropharyngeal structures, obstruction of the upper gastrointestinal tract, and/or xerostomia.[20] However, dysphagia may be related to other factors, e.g. mucosal inflammation.[21]

Dysphagia is associated with significant morbidity. The direct effects of dysphagia include dehydration, malnutrition, and weight loss. Dysphagia may also be associated with drooling of saliva, and aspiration of food/drink. The indirect effects of dysphagia include other physical problems (e.g. fatigue), as well as psychological problems (e.g. depression). Indeed, dysphagia/nutritional problems have a significant impact on quality of life in this group of patients.

The management of dysphagia involves:[20,21]

◆ Treatment of underlying cause.

◆ Swallowing therapy – use of different postures when swallowing, and different techniques of swallowing.

◆ Swallowing aids – adaptation of normal utensils (e.g. cups), and production of specific aids (e.g. intra-oral prostheses).

◆ Dietary manipulation – use of differing volumes of food, and differing consistencies of food.

◆ Nasogastric (NG) feeding.

◆ Percutaneous endoscopic gastrostomy (PEG) feeding.

The decision to initiate non-oral feeding depends on a number of factors, including the cause of dysphagia (irreversible, reversible), the response to other interventions, the patient's symptomatology (hungry, not hungry), and the patient's prognosis.[21] In general, nasogastric feeding is used for short-term feeding (days to weeks), whilst PEG feeding is used for longer-term feeding (weeks to months).[21]

Other factors associated with nutritional problems include anorexia, taste disturbance, oral discomfort, inadequate dentition (missing teeth), inadequate dentures (loose dentures), alcohol dependence (poor diet) and social isolation (poor diet). It should be noted that many of these factors are amenable to relatively simple interventions, e.g. loose dentures may be replaced or relined.

A dietician should review patients with nutritional problems, whilst a speech and language therapist should also review patients with dysphagia.

Communication problems

Communication problems are common in patients with head and neck cancer. For example, the reported prevalence is 30–53 per cent amongst patients with advanced head and neck cancer.[9,15]

Communication problems are invariably related to damage to relevant structures in the head and neck region.[16] Other contributory factors include xerostomia, dental problems (missing teeth), denture problems (loose dentures) and deafness.[16]

The management of the communication problem depends on the aetiology of the communication problem. Specific interventions include the use of artificial larynx vibrators and Blom–Singer valves.[22] Non-specific interventions include the use of 'low-tech' communication aids (e.g. picture boards), and 'high-tech' communication aids (e.g. electronic keyboards).[23] A speech and language therapist should review all patients with communication problems.

Tumour/wound problems

Fungation

Fungation is reported to occur in 14–15 per cent patients with advanced disease.[10,15] In some cases, specific treatment may be indicated (i.e. radiotherapy, surgery). However, in the majority of cases, the management is conservative. Management consists of routine hygiene measures, use of appropriate wound products/dressings, treatment of malodour (wound products, antibiotics), protection of surrounding skin (barrier creams) and treatment of associated symptoms.[24]

Fistula

Cutaneous fistulae are reported to occur in 21 per cent patients with advanced disease.[9] The management of a fistula is very similar to the management of fungation. In some cases, specific treatment may be indicated (i.e. surgery). However, in the majority of cases, the management is conservative. Management consists of routine hygiene measures, collection of effluent (wound products, stoma devices), protection of surrounding skin (barrier creams) and treatment of associated symptoms.[24] Large defects may be filled with an absorbent material and covered with a waterproof dressing (Figs 14.2(a)–(c).

Bleeding

Minor haemorrhages are relatively common (reported prevalence 18–47 per cent).[9,10] However, major haemorrhages are much less common.[15] Moreover, major haemorrhages are a relatively unusual cause of death in this group of patients (see below).[9,10]

The management of haemorrhage depends on a number of factors, including the patient's general condition, the cause of the bleeding, the severity of the bleeding, and the sequelae of the bleeding.[25] It is important that a management plan is developed for patients at risk of haemorrhage. It is equally important that the management plan is reassessed on a regular basis.

The acute management of minor/non-threatening bleeding may involve the use of local pressure, haemostatic dressings (e.g. alginate), topical vasoconstrictors (e.g. epinephrine), topical astringents (e.g. sucralfate), topical haemostatic agents (e.g. tranexamic acid), cauterising agents (e.g. silver nitrate) and systemic haemostatic agents (e.g. tranexamic acid).[25,26] It is also important to correct any associated haemostatic problems, e.g. reverse anticoagulation.

Subsequently, some patients may be suitable for specific interventions aimed at preventing further bleeding, e.g. radiotherapy, embolization.[25] In addition, patients with symptomatic anaemia may benefit from the administration of haematinics and/or a blood transfusion.

The acute management of major or life-threatening bleeding should involve the use of sedative drugs (e.g. midazolam).[27] In most cases, a subcutaneous injection of 10 mg of midazolam will adequately sedate the patient. However, some patients require

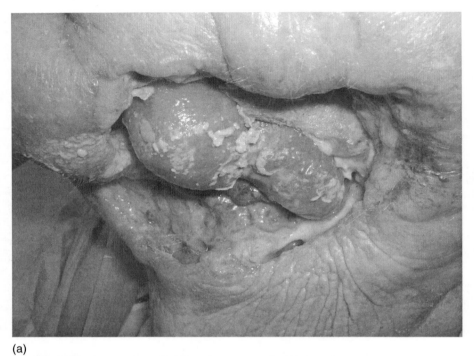

(a)

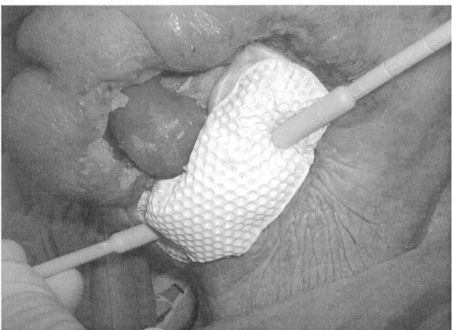

(b)

Fig. 14.2 Conservative management of large orocutaneous fistula.

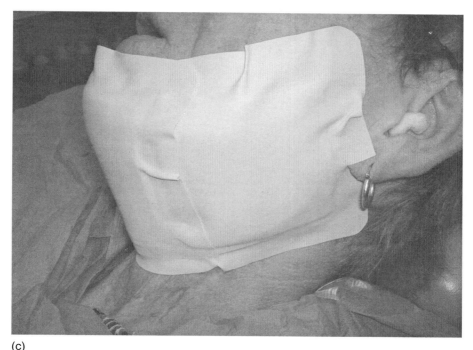

(c)

Fig. 14.2 Cont'd

further/larger doses of midazolam, e.g. patients on long-term benzodiazepine therapy. The appropriate use of midazolam does not negatively influence the outcome of the bleeding event.

Major bleeds are generally preceded by minor ('herald') bleeds. Thus, it may be possible to identify 'at risk' patients, and make preparations for such an eventuality. In such circumstances, it is recommended that the sedative drug, and other relevant items (pressure dressings, coloured blankets), are kept in close proximity to the patient.[27]

Other physical problems

Patients with head and neck cancer may experience a variety of oral symptoms, including xerostomia, taste disturbance and halitosis. These oral symptoms are discussed in detail in Chapters 9–11. Patients with head and neck cancer may also experience a variety of systemic symptoms, e.g. nausea and vomiting, constipation.[11] Indeed, patients often report a number of contemporaneous symptoms/problems.[9]

Psychosocial problems

Psychological problems (anxiety, depression) are common in patients with cancer, but appear to be particularly common in patients with head and neck cancer.[28] For example,

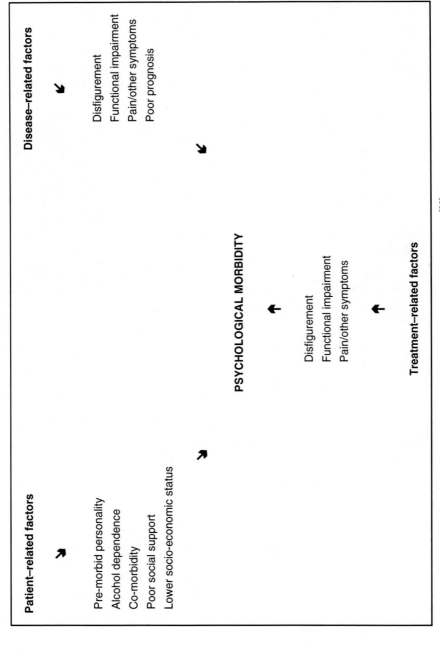

Fig. 14.3 Factors associated with psychological morbidity in patients with head and neck cancer.[28]

one study reported a prevalence of depression of 40 per cent amongst a mixed group of patients with head and neck cancer.[29]

Psychological problems may occur at any stage of the disease (i.e. at diagnosis, during treatment, during remission, at relapse). However, psychological problems are especially common in advanced disease.[28] It should be noted that patients with head and neck cancer are at an increased risk of suicide.[28]

The factors associated with psychological morbidity in patients with head and neck cancer are shown in Fig. 14.3. Many of these factors are generic, but some are relatively specific to patients with head and neck cancer (e.g. facial disfigurement). Interestingly, studies suggest that certain generic factors are particularly important in this group of patients (e.g. poor social support).[29]

Other psychosocial consequences of head and neck cancer include altered body image, loss of identity, loss of confidence, relationship problems and psychosexual problems.[2,30] Moreover, patients may avoid all types of social interaction, including forfeiting relationships, friendships, employment, hobbies and other social activities.

Patients with these problems should be reviewed by appropriate members of the extended multidisciplinary team, e.g. clinical psychologist, social worker.

The terminal phase

In most instances, patients die as a result of gradual deterioration in their condition.[9,10] Furthermore, the majority of patients have a relatively uneventful terminal phase.[9] Nevertheless, in some instances, patients die as a result of an acute complication of their disease, e.g. haemorrhage, airway obstruction. Table 14.1 demonstrates the cause of death amongst a cohort of patients with head and neck cancer admitted to a hospice in the United Kingdom.[9]

Table 14.1 Causes of death in head and neck patients receiving palliative care[9]

Cause of death	Number of patients $N = 36$ (%)
Progressive disease*	17 (47)
Bronchopneumonia	9 (25)
Massive haemorrhage	3 (8)
Airway obstruction	2 (6)
Myocardial infarction	2 (6)
Cardiac failure	2 (6)
Other	1 (2)

* Condition gradually deteriorated

References

1. Rhys Evans PH, Patel SG (2003). Introduction. In PH Rhys Evans, PQ Montgomery, PJ Gullane (ed.). *Principles and Practice of Head and Neck Oncology*, pp. 3–13. London: Martin Dunitz.

2. Fardy M (1997). Oro-facial cancer – is there more to treatment than surgery and radiotherapy? *Palliative Care Today* 6: 20–1.

3. Rhys Evans PH, Montgomery PQ, Gullane PJ (2003). *Principles and Practice of Head and Neck Oncology*. London: Martin Dunitz.

4. Souhami RL, Tannock I, Hohenberger P, Horiot J-C (2002). *Oxford Textbook of Oncology*, 2nd edn. Oxford: Oxford University Press.

5. Wood RE (2003). Dental management of the head and neck cancer patient. In PH Rhys Evans, PQ Montgomery, PJ Gullane (ed.). *Principles and Practice of Head and Neck Oncology*, pp. 137–48. London: Martin Dunitz.

6. Curran AJ, Irish JC, Gullane PJ (2003). Complications in head and neck cancer surgery. In PH Rhys Evans, PQ Montgomery, PJ Gullane (ed.). *Principles and Practice of Head and Neck Oncology*, pp. 487–501. London: Martin Dunitz.

7. Henk JM (2003). Principles of head and neck radiotherapy. In PH Rhys Evans, PQ Montgomery, PJ Gullane (ed.). *Principles and Practice of Head and Neck Oncology*, pp. 65–78. London: Martin Dunitz.

8. Saini A, Gore ME, Adelstein DJ (2003). Chemotherapy for head and neck cancer. In PH Rhys Evans, PQ Montgomery, PJ Gullane (ed.). *Principles and Practice of Head and Neck Oncology*, pp. 79–98. London: Martin Dunitz.

9. Forbes K (1997). Palliative care in patients with cancer of the head and neck. *Clin Otolaryngol* 22: 117–22.

10. Shedd DP, Carl A, Shedd C (1980). Problems of terminal head and neck cancer patients. *Head Neck Surg* 2: 476–82.

11. Grond S, Zech D, Lynch J, Diefenbach C, Schug SA, Lehmann KA (1993). Validation of World Health Organization guidelines for pain relief in head and neck cancer. A prospective study. *Ann Otol Rhinol Laryngol* 102: 342–8.

12. World Health Organization (1996). *Cancer Pain Relief*, 2nd edn. Geneva: WHO.

13. Varghese BT, Koshy RC, Sebastian P, Joseph E (2002). Combined sphenopalatine ganglion and mandibular nerve, neurolytic block for pain due to advanced head and neck cancer. *Palliat Med* 16: 447–8.

14. Wall PD, Melzack R (1999). *Textbook of Pain*, 4th edn. Edinburgh: Churchill Livingstone.

15. Aird DW, Bihari J, Smith C (1983). Clinical problems in the continuing care of head and neck cancer patients. *Ear Nose Throat J* 62: 230–43.

16. Murphy BA, Cmelak A, Bayles S, Dowling E, Billante CR (2003). In D Doyle, G Hanks, N Cherny, K Calman (ed.) *Oxford Textbook of Palliative Medicine*, 3rd edn, pp. 658–73. Oxford: Oxford University Press.

17. Biller JA (2002). Airway obstruction, bronchospasm, and cough. In AM Berger, RK Portenoy, DE Weissman (ed.) *Principles and Practice of Palliative Care and Supportive Oncology*, 2nd edn, pp. 378–88. Philadelphia: Lippincott Williams & Wilkins.

18. Chan K-S, Sham MM, Tse DM, Thorsen AB (2003). Palliative medicine in malignant respiratory diseases. In D Doyle, G Hanks, N Cherny, K Calman (ed.) *Oxford Textbook of Palliative Medicine*, 3rd edn, pp. 587–618. Oxford: Oxford University Press.

19. Regnard C, Hockley J (2004). *A Guide to Symptom Relief in Palliative Care*. Oxford: Radcliffe Medical Press.

20. Leder SB (2002). Dysphagia. In AM Berger, RK Portenoy, DE Weissman (ed.) *Principles and Practice of Palliative Care and Supportive Oncology*, 2nd edn, pp. 194–205. Philadelphia: Lippincott Williams & Wilkins.

21. Regnard C (2003). Dysphagia, dyspepsia, and hiccup. In D Doyle, G Hanks, N Cherny, K Calman (ed.) *Oxford Textbook of Palliative Medicine*, 3rd edn, pp. 468–83. Oxford: Oxford University Press.

22. Rhys Evans PH, Blom ED (2003). Functional restoration of speech. In PH Rhys Evans, PQ Montgomery, PJ Gullane (ed.). *Principles and Practice of Head and Neck Oncology*, pp. 571–602. London: Martin Dunitz.

23. MacDonald A, Armstrong L (2003). The contribution of speech and language therapy to palliative medicine. In D Doyle, G Hanks, N Cherny, K Calman (ed.) *Oxford Textbook of Palliative Medicine*, 3rd edn, pp. 1057–63. Oxford: Oxford University Press.

24. Grocott P, Dealey C (2003). Skin problems in palliative medicine: nursing aspects. In D Doyle, G Hanks, N Cherny, K Calman (ed.) *Oxford Textbook of Palliative Medicine*, 3rd edn, pp. 628–40. Oxford: Oxford University Press.

25. Friedman KD, Raife TJ (2002). Management of hypercoagulable states and coagulopathy. In AM Berger, RK Portenoy, DE Weissman (ed.) *Principles and Practice of Palliative Care and Supportive Oncology*, 2nd edn, pp. 452–62. Philadelphia: Lippincott Williams & Wilkins.

26. Twycross R, Wilcock A (2001). *Symptom Management in Advanced Cancer*, 3rd edn, pp. 237–8. Oxford: Radcliffe Medical Press.

27. Lovel T (2000). Palliative care and head and neck cancer. *Br J Oral Maxillofac Surg* 38: 253–4.

28. Frampton M (2001). Psychological distress in patients with head and neck cancer: review. *Br J Oral Maxillofac Surg* 39: 67–70.

29. Baile WF, Gilbertini M, Scott L, Endicott J (1992). Depression and tumour stage in cancer of the head and neck. *Psychooncology* 1: 15–24.

30. Gamba A, Romano M, Grosso IM, Tamburini M, Cantu G, Molinari R *et al.* (1992). Psychosocial adjustment of patients surgically treated for head and neck cancer. *Head Neck* 14: 218–23.

Chapter 15

Oral complications of cancer treatment

Mark Chambers, Adam Garden, James Lemon, Merrill Kies and Jack Martin

Introduction

Cancer therapy can cause complex oral and dental complications. The complications vary by patient, and depend on the individual's baseline oral and dental status, the type of cancer, and the type of cancer therapy being administered.[1] In most cases, pre-existing conditions strongly influence the development of complications in the oral cavity.[1] The oral complications associated with chemotherapy are shown in Table 15.1,[2] whilst those associated with head and neck radiation therapy are shown in Table 15.2.[2]

Oral mucosal and dental sequelae cause significant morbidity, can produce fatal events (e.g. oral infection leading to systemic infection) and can compromise treatment, (e.g. oral mucositis leading to treatment being delayed, decreased, or even discontinued).[2] It should be noted that any compromise of a treatment regimen might decrease the success of that treatment regimen with regard to controlling disease. Nevertheless, oral complications can be minimized, and in some cases eliminated, if identified and addressed early by the multidisciplinary team.

This chapter describes the oral complications that can result from chemotherapy and head and neck radiation therapy, and presents a philosophy for preventing and treating such complications.

Generic issues

Pretreatment assessment

Physicians have a responsibility to ensure that patients with cancer who receive chemotherapy, head and neck radiation therapy, or any combination of these treatments first receive a thorough and systematic oral examination.[3] The goals of the initial examination are to identify any pre-existing pathologic conditions that might impact the cancer treatment plan (e.g. dental caries, periodontal disease, partially erupted teeth, soft-tissue trauma).[3]

Table 15.1 Oral complications of chemotherapy[2]

Complication	Comment
Oral mucositis	Acute complication – see text
Oral infections – viral – fungal – bacterial	Acute complication – see text
Haemorrhage	Acute complication Haemorrhage may occur with oral mucositis, oral infections and/or thrombocytopenia
Oral pain	Acute complication Pain in the mandible may occur with vinca alkaloids
Taste disturbance	Acute complication – see Chapter 10
Salivary gland dysfunction	Acute complication – see text
Induction of second malignancy	Chronic complication

A head and neck evaluation, oral and dental clinical examination, and intra-oral radiologic evaluation should all be performed.[3] Selected dental radiographs are essential in evaluating potential problems that are not obvious on clinical examination (e.g. periodontal/periapical tooth pathology, impacted teeth, partially erupted teeth). The patient's ability to maintain optimal oral hygiene should also be evaluated during the initial examination.[4]

The dental specialist should communicate with the treating oncologist to find out the diagnosis and stage of the malignant disease, the patient's prognosis, the type of

Table 15.2 Oral complications of head and neck radiation therapy[2]

Complication	Comment
Oral mucositis	Acute complication – see text
Oral infections – fungal – bacterial	Acute/chronic complication – see text
Taste disturbance	Acute/chronic complication – see Chapter 10
Salivary gland dysfunction	Acute/chronic complication – see text
Osteoradionecrosis	Chronic complication – see text
Soft tissue necrosis	Chronic complication (cf. osteoradionecrosis)
Soft tissue fibrosis	Chronic complication Trismus may result from fibrosis of the muscles of mastication and/or the temporomandibular joint
Induction of second malignancy	Chronic complication

treatment, the goals of treatment, and any other relevant medical details. These factors will help the dentist determine what preventive or treatment steps to take to manage complications. The patient's medical and haematologic status must be reviewed with the treating oncologist before initiating any such dental treatment.[5]

Pretreatment management

Any potential source of oral infection should be eliminated. Extractions and associated alveoloplasty should be performed as atraumatically as possible, and should include smoothing of surrounding hard tissue, appropriate irrigation and attempts at primary closure in order to promote rapid healing.[6] To ensure adequate wound healing, extractions should be performed 2–3 weeks before initiation of cancer therapy.[7]

Oral treatment plans should also be designed to correct restoration overhangs, rough or edges on teeth, and any other defects likely to cause soft-tissue irritation.[8] Dental implants should be carefully assessed, and their removal should be considered if integration is poor, or if maintenance of peri-implant health cannot be anticipated. Ill-fitting intra-oral prostheses should not be worn during cancer therapy.

Periodontal procedures such as scaling and root planning may be necessary before cancer treatment to reduce the oral bacterial load. Daily plaque removal procedures should be emphasized, including brushing with a fluoride toothpaste and flossing. Oral hygiene procedures may require modification during cancer therapy (see below).

Dental specialists should educate patients who use tobacco, alcohol, or illicit drugs about the physical effects of these substances, and their potential effect on treatment outcome.[9] For example, smoking and drinking alcohol can aggravate oral mucositis.

The patient's nutritional status should be assessed, and nutritional counselling should be provided, if needed, to help patients understand that a healthy diet is important for avoiding debilitation, delayed wound healing, and increased susceptibility to dental caries.[10] Patients should be instructed to avoid abrasive foods likely to traumatize soft tissues during treatment.

Some oncology centres perform microbiologic cultures, with appropriate sensitivity testing, to assess herpes simplex virus antibody titres, fungal activity and bacterial activity. In cases of positive results, prophylactic use of an antiviral agent such as aciclovir, an antifungal agent such as nystatin, or an antimicrobial agent such as clindamycin is employed.

It is important to note that treatment of the cancer must always take priority over treatment of any oral and dental problems.[3]

Ongoing management

Care should be focused on the prevention of complications, by eliminating known factors that initiate pathology and promoting good hygiene, hydration and nutrition.

Oral hygiene procedures may require modification during cancer therapy, e.g. using a very soft-bristled toothbrush. The fear that brushing will increase the chances of oral complications has always been a concern for practitioners, yet the benefits of brushing outweigh the drawbacks. The use of oral rinses to control plaque is a poor substitute for brushing.

The daily use of topically applied fluorides, and sodium bicarbonate or chlorhexidine gluconate mouth rinses, will reduce bacterial and fungal contamination.[11,12] The mouth rinse prescribed should be carefully selected, because some ingredients, such as alcohol and phenol, are caustic to oral mucosal tissues.

The National Cancer Institute (United States of America) has developed guidelines for the prevention/management of the oral complications of chemotherapy and head and neck radiation therapy.[2] These guidelines are reviewed on a regular basis, and updated as necessary.

Specific problems

Oral mucositis

Mucositis is defined as 'inflammation of a mucous surface'.[13] The term oral mucositis is generally used to describe inflammation secondary to chemotherapy, or head and neck radiation therapy. The term oral stomatitis is used to describe inflammation secondary to other causes, e.g. infection, trauma.

Epidemiology

Oral mucositis is a common acute complication of chemotherapy and head and neck radiation therapy. Indeed, approximately 40 per cent of patients who receive standard chemotherapy, and almost all patients who receive head and neck radiation therapy, develop some degree of oral mucositis.[14]

The prevalence of oral mucositis is affected by a number of factors, including the patient's age (more common in the young), diagnosis (increased in patients with haematological malignancy), and pre-existing oral health (increased in patients with poor oral health).[15]

Aetiology

Sonis has proposed a four-phase model to explain the pathophysiology of oral mucositis[15]:

1. Inflammatory/vascular phase
2. Epithelial phase
3. Ulcerative/bacteriological phase
4. Healing phase.

Inflammatory/vascular phase   Chemotherapy and radiation therapy stimulate the release of cytokines from epithelial cells (i.e. tumour necrosis factor α, interleukin 1).

In addition, radiation therapy stimulates the release of cytokines from adjacent connective tissue. Tumour necrosis factor α causes local tissue damage, whilst interleukin 1 causes localized inflammation (increased vascularity).

Epithelial phase   Chemotherapy and radiation therapy suppress dividing cells in the basal layer of the epithelium, which affects the regeneration of cells in the upper layers of the epithelium. As a consequence, the epithelium becomes thinned, and then ulcerated. Ulceration is exacerbated by the continued release of cytokines, and by 'functional' trauma (e.g. eating).

Ulcerative/bacteriological phase   This phase is characterized by ulceration of the epithelium. The ulcers become colonized with Gram-negative bacteria that produce endotoxins, which stimulate the release of cytokines and the production of nitric oxide. The cytokines and nitric acid cause further local tissue damage and localized inflammation.

Healing phase   This phase is characterized by regeneration of the epithelium.

Considerable inter-patient variability exists in the tolerance to chemotherapy regimens.[16] Treatment factors that influence the frequency and severity of oral mucositis include the chemotherapeutic agent used, dosage, delivery schedule, and combination with radiation therapy.[17]

The severity of radiation-induced mucositis also depends on a number of factors, including total dose, dose fractionation, volume of tissue irradiated and type of radiation given.[17]

Other factors that may contribute to the severity of mucositis include smoking, use of over-the-counter mouthwashes and coexistence of collagen vascular diseases or HIV infection.[17]

Clinical features

The most consistent symptom of mucositis is pain. The severity of pain correlates with the severity of the mucositis.[18] The pain is constant in nature, and is aggravated by drinking, eating, and performance of oral hygiene measures (see below).

All intra-oral sites may be affected, although non-keratinized surfaces are most severely affected (mucosa of lips, cheeks, floor of mouth, ventral surface of tongue, and soft palate). Erythema is the initial manifestation, followed by the development of white desquamative patches. Epithelial sloughing and fibrinous exudate lead to the formation of ulceration and a pseudomembrane (Fig. 15.1).[17]

A number of grading systems for oral mucositis have been developed.[17] However, to date, no grading scale has been universally accepted. One commonly used grading scale is the National Cancer Institute's Common Toxicity Criteria scale (Table 15.3).[19]

The complications of oral mucositis include dehydration, malnutrition, local infection, systemic infection, local haemorrhage, and interference with the cancer treatment regimen. The latter complication is particularly important, since a delay in completing treatment, or a reduction in the amount of treatment given, may influence the eventual outcome of treatment.

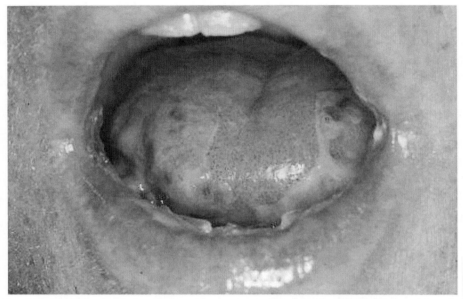

Fig. 15.1 Chemotherapy-induced mucositis. Courtesy of M Chambers. (See also Plate 32 at the centre of this book.)

Oral mucositis is a self-limiting condition, with recovery occurring around two weeks after a course of chemotherapy, and approximately 3–4 weeks after a course of radiation therapy.[20] Preexisting or predisposing factors that challenge wound healing can affect recovery from oral mucositis (e.g. infection).[15]

Management

There is no standard therapy that is effective in the prevention of oral mucositis. The range of medications that have been used is extensive. A recent systematic review identified 21 interventions that had been subjected to randomized controlled trials, but found evidence of benefit for only nine of these interventions.[21] The authors

Table 15.3 National Cancer Institute CTC mucositis scoring system[19]

Grade	Clinical features
0	None
1	Painless ulcers, erythema or mild soreness
2	Painful erythema, oedema, or ulcers, can eat
3	Painful erythema, oedema, or ulcers, cannot eat
4	Requires parenteral or enteral support

concluded that there was some ('sometimes weak') evidence to support the use of allopurinol, amifostine, antibiotics, GM-CSF, hydrolytic enzymes, ice chips, povidone and oral care. In many instances, the evidence for the effectiveness of the intervention was based on studies performed in specific patient or treatment groups. For example, the studies showing benefit from the use of ice chips were performed in patients receiving bolus 5-FU chemotherapy.

Similarly, there is no standard therapy that is effective in the treatment/reversal of oral mucositis. A recent systematic review identified six interventions that had been subjected to randomized controlled trials, but found evidence of benefit for only two of these interventions.[22] The authors concluded that there was weak ('unreliable') evidence to support the use of allopurinol mouthwash and vitamin E. Thus, the major objective in the treatment of mucositis is palliation.

The mainstay of the symptomatic management of oral mucositis is the use of analgesics. In some cases, topical analgesics will control the pain (see Chapter 12). Nevertheless, in many cases, topical analgesics need to be supplemented or replaced by systemic analgesics. The principles of pain relief in this condition are the same as the general principles of pain relief in patients with cancer.[23] Patients often require opioids for moderate to severe pain ('strong' opioids) to control their pain, and often these opioids need to be given by parenteral administration.

Salivary gland dysfunction

Epidemiology

Salivary gland dysfunction (SGD) is a common problem in patients with cancer.

Aetiology

Salivary gland dysfunction may result from a reduction in salivary flow and/or an alteration of salivary composition.

The most common cause for salivary gland dysfunction is drug treatment. Several drugs can produce SGD, including chemotherapy agents (e.g. busulfan, procarbazine) and supportive care agents (e.g. analgesics, antiemetics).[24] Drug-induced SGD is generally reversible, i.e. discontinuation of the drug leads to resolution of the problem.

Salivary gland dysfunction is a predictable side-effect of radiation therapy to the head and neck region.[25] It also occurs in patients that receive total body irradiation as part of the conditioning regimen for a bone marrow transplant. Radiation-induced SGD is generally irreversible. The severity of radiation-induced SGD is influenced by both radiation therapy regimen (field, dose) and pretreatment salivary gland function.[25]

Clinical features

Individuals with SGD can exhibit innumerable problems, including xerostomia, oral discomfort, taste disturbance, difficulty chewing, difficulty swallowing, difficulty speaking, dental caries and other oral infections. Salivary gland dysfunction may also intensify, or prolong, the process of oral mucositis.[26] These problems reflect the major functional roles of saliva.

Management

Various strategies have been employed to try to reduce the impact of radiation therapy on salivary gland function, including salivary gland shielding,[25] use of radioprotectors (amifostine),[27] use of parasympathomimetic drugs (pilocarpine)[28] and use of parasympatholytic drugs (biperiden).[29] The Oral Heath Group of the Cochrane Collaboration is in the process of undertaking a systematic review of the efficacy of these interventions (Dr Andrew Davies, personal communication).

Similarly, various strategies have been employed to overcome SGD, and to manage the sequelae of SGD. Selection of an adequate management regimen for a particular patient with xerostomia should be based on general clinical criteria: subjective discomfort, presence of oral changes and presence of any additional factors that compromise oral health.[3] The options for treating SGD include the use of saliva stimulants, saliva substitutes, or a combination of both.[30]

Initially, treatment is aimed at restoring the flow of saliva, i.e. use of saliva stimulants. Pilocarpine has been shown to be effective in the management of SGD secondary to radiation therapy. Approximately 50 per cent of patients report an improvement in symptoms, although many develop related side-effects (e.g. sweating, urinary frequency).[31,32] Other cholinergic agonists may also be useful in this setting. Acupuncture has also been reported to be effective in the management of SGD secondary to radiation therapy.[33] However, there is relatively little evidence to support the use of other salivary stimulants in this setting (e.g. chewing gum, organic acids).

However, if the flow of saliva cannot be restored, then saliva substitutes should be used (e.g. artificial salivas, other agents). Most saliva substitutes provide only short-term relief of symptoms, and they can irritate the already sensitive oral tissues.[34] In addition, if the flow of saliva cannot be restored, then the daily use of fluoride is necessary to prevent dental caries.

Salivary gland dysfunction is discussed in detail in Chapter 9.

Osteoradionecrosis

Osteoradionecrosis (ORN) has been defined as 'radiological evidence of bone necrosis within the radiation field, where tumour recurrence has been excluded'.[35]

Epidemiology

Osteoradionecrosis has become a relatively uncommon chronic complication of head and neck radiation therapy.[36] The reasons for the decline in the incidence of ORN include improvements in radiation therapy (megavoltage therapy) and improvements in supportive care (oral/dental care).

Aetiology

The underlying mechanisms of ORN relate to the 'three H principle' of irradiated tissue, i.e. hypocellularity, hypovascularity, and hypoxia. In such tissue, the ability to replace normal cellular and collagen loss is severely compromised, with resultant necrosis occurring in relation to the rate of normal or induced cellular death and collagen lysis.[37] The risk of ORN following trauma or oral surgical procedures can be highly significant.

Osteoradionecrosis has been associated with a number of different factors,[36] including:

- Patient-related factors – poor oral hygiene, dental extractions (post radiation therapy)
- Disease-related factors – tumor size, tumour location
- Radiation therapy-related factors – radiation dose, radiation fractionation.

Clinical features

Osteoradionecrosis may occur at any time following radiation therapy, but commonly occurs within three years of the radiation therapy.[36] The mandible is much more susceptible to osteoradionecrosis than the maxilla. The clinical features are influenced by the stage of the process. Patients with early stage ORN may be relatively asymptomatic. In contrast, patients with advanced stage ORN are often very symptomatic (pain, discharge).

Store *et al.* have proposed the following classification of osteoradionecrosis:[35]

- Stage 0 – exposed bone; no radiological signs
- Stage 1 – mucosa intact; radiological signs present
- Stage 2 – exposed bone; radiological signs present
- Stage 3 – exposed bone; radiological signs present; orocutaneous fistula; localized infection (Fig. 15.2).

It should be noted that patients with stage 0 disease do not fulfill the aforementioned definition of osteoradionecrosis. However, patients with stage 0 disease often progress to stage 2 disease.[35] Indeed, the stage of the disease frequently changes, and may improve as well as deteriorate.[35]

The diagnosis of osteoradionecrosis is based on a combination of clinical features and radiological features.[36] Plain X-rays show decreased bone density, and may show fractures. CT scans show bone abnormalities such as focal lytic areas, cortical breaks, and loss of spongiosa trabeculation (Fig. 15.3). Other imaging techniques will also show bone abnormalities (i.e. bone scanning, MRI).

Management

The most important aspect of management is prevention. Osteoradionecrosis may be avoided if patients receive appropriate dental care prior to radiation therapy, maintain

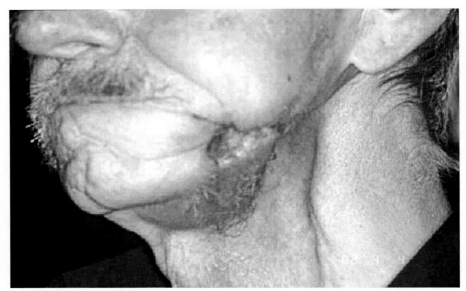

Fig. 15.2 Osteoradionecrosis. Courtesy of MP Sweeney. (See also Plate 33 at the centre of this book.)

high standards of oral hygiene during/post radiation therapy, and avoid dental extractions and other types of oral surgery post radiation therapy.

If oral surgical intervention is required after radiation therapy, then pre- and post-operative hyperbaric oxygen therapy may increase the potential for healing, while minimizing the risk for ORN.[38] Hyperbaric oxygen therapy increases wound healing capacity by stimulating osteogenesis and angiogenesis. It should be noted that many dental procedures can be safely done after radiation therapy, including routine restorative procedures, endodontic procedures and prosthetic procedures.

In most cases, the management of ORN is conservative, and involves some or all of the following modalities: removal of loose bone fragments, gentle sequestration, irrigation, topical antiseptics, systemic antibiotics and/or hyperbaric oxygen.[36] Other modalities that have been reported to be effective include pentoxyphilline and vitamin E, ultrasound therapy, and electromagnetic stimulation.[36] In advanced (symptomatic) cases, the management of ORN is surgical, and involves either radical sequestration, or hemimandibulectomy with reconstruction.[39,40]

Oral infections

Oral infections are a common acute complication of chemotherapy. A variety of different infections may occur, particularly fungal (oral candidosis) and viral (e.g. herpes simplex virus) infections. The aetiology of these infections includes damage to the oral mucosa and systemic immunosuppression.[14] Oral infections usually occur in

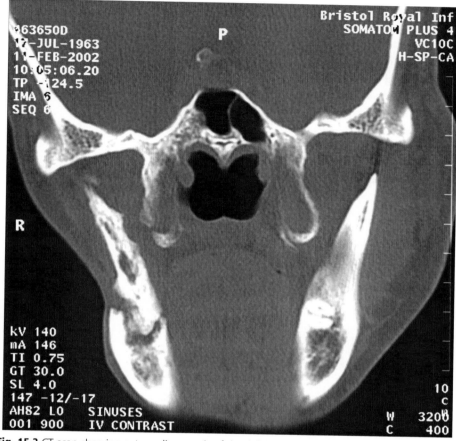

Fig. 15.3 CT scan showing osteoradionecrosis of the right mandible. Courtesy of Dr Julian Kabala.

association with the haematological nadir, although they may occur at other times in the chemotherapy cycle. For example, oral herpes simplex virus infections can be seen early in the chemotherapy cycle.

Similarly, oral infections are a common acute/chronic complication of head and neck radiation therapy. A variety of different infections may occur, particularly fungal (oral candidosis) and bacterial (e.g. dental caries) infections. The aetiology of these infections includes damage to the oral mucosa and salivary gland dysfunction.[14] The chronic nature of these infections reflects the ongoing nature of the salivary gland dysfunction. Fig. 7.2 shows an example of dental caries in a patient with radiation-induced salivary gland dysfunction.

Oral infections can cause morbidity per se, can aggravate oral mucositis, and can lead to systemic infections. The clinical features may be relatively specific, or relatively non-specific (such as oral mucositis). Moreover, the clinical features may be typical, or, particularly in immunosuppressed patients, atypical. Figures 8.3 and 8.4 show examples of atypical herpes simplex virus infections. Thus, healthcare professionals should have a low threshold for screening for the presence of such oral infections.

Systemic infections are also a relatively common acute complication of chemotherapy. As discussed above, the oral cavity is often the primary source of the offending organisms.[41,42] Systemic infections can be life threatening, and so it is important that oral infections are recognized, properly diagnosed and aggressively treated.

Oral infections are discussed in detail in Chapters 6–8.

References

1. Toth BB, Martin JW, Fleming TJ (1991). Oral and dental care associated with cancer therapy. *Cancer Bull* **43**: 397–402.
2. National Cancer Institute (2004). *Oral Complications of Chemotherapy and Head/Neck Radiation Monograph on the Internet.* Bethesda: NCI, Available from: http://www.cancer.gov/cancerinfo/pdq/supportivecare/oralcomplications/HealthProfessional
3. Chambers MS, Toth BB, Martin JW, Fleming TJ, Lemon JC (1995). Oral and dental management of the cancer patient: prevention and treatment of complications. *Support Care Cancer* **3**: 168–75.
4. Lindquist SF, Hickey AJ, Drane JB (1978). Effect of oral hygiene on stomatitis in patients receiving cancer chemotherapy. *J Prosthet Dent* **40**: 312–14.
5. King GE, Lemon JC, Martin JW (1992). Multidisciplinary teamwork in the treatment and rehabilitation of the head and neck cancer patient. *Texas Dent J* **109**: 9–12.
6. Westcott WB (1985). Dental management of patients being treated for oral cancer. *CDA J* **13**: 42–7.
7. Peterson DE (1983). Dental care for the cancer patient. *Compend Contin Educ Dent* **4**: 115–20.
8. Engelmeier RL (1987). A dental protocol for patients receiving radiation therapy for cancer of the head and neck. *Spec Care Dentist* **7**: 54–8.
9. Toth BB, Chambers MS, Fleming TJ, Lemon JC, Martin JW (1995). Minimizing oral complications of cancer treatment. *Oncology* **9**: 851–8.
10. Guo CB, Ma DQ, Zhang KH (1994). Applicability of the general nutritional status score to patients with oral and maxillofacial malignancies. *Int J Oral Maxillofac Surg* **23**: 167–9.
11. Toth BB, Martin JW, Fleming TJ (1990). Oral complications associated with cancer therapy: An M. D. Anderson Cancer Center experience. *J Clin Periodontol* **17**: 508–15.
12. Ciancio S (1994). Expanded and future uses of mouthrinses. *J Am Dent Assoc* **125**, Suppl 2: 29S–32S.
13. Critchley M (1978). *Butterworths Medical Dictionary*, 2nd edn. London: Butterworths.
14. Scully C, Epstein JB (1996). Oral health care for the cancer patient. *Eur J Cancer B Oral Oncol* **32B**: 281–92.
15. Sonis ST (1998). Mucositis as a biological process: a new hypothesis for the development of chemotherapy-induced stomatotoxicity. *Oral Oncol* **34**: 39–43.
16. Sonis S, Clark J (1991). Prevention and management of oral mucositis induced by antineoplastic therapy. *Oncol (Huntingt)* **5**: 11–18.
17. Parulekar W, Mackenzie R, Bjarnason G, Jordan RC (1998). Scoring oral mucositis. *Oral Oncol* **34**: 63–71.

18. Sonis ST, Eilers JP, Epstein JB, LeVeque FG, Liggett WH Jr, Mulagha MT *et al.* (1999). Validation of a new scoring system for the assessment of the clinical trial research of oral mucositis induced by radiation or chemotherapy. *Cancer* **85**: 2103–13.

19. Anonymous (1989). Oral complications of cancer therapies: diagnosis, prevention and treatment. National Institutes of Health. *Conn Med* **53**: 595–601.

20. Sonis ST, Fazio RC, Fang L (1984). *Principles and Practice of Oral Medicine.* Philadelphia: W B Saunders Company.

21. Clarkson JE, Worthington HV, Eden OB (2003). *Interventions for Preventing Oral Mucositis for Patients with Cancer Receiving Treatment* (Cochrane Review). In The Cochrane Library, Issue 4. Chichester, UK: John Wiley & Sons Ltd.

22. Worthington HV, Clarkson JE, Eden OB (2003). *Interventions for Treating Oral Mucositis for Patients with Cancer Receiving Treatment* (Cochrane Review). In The Cochrane Library, Issue 4. Chichester, UK: John Wiley & Sons Ltd.

23. World Health Organization (1996). *Cancer Pain Relief,* 2nd edn. Geneva: WHO.

24. Sreebny LM, Schwartz SS (1997). A reference guide to drugs and dry mouth-2nd edn. *Gerodontology* **14**: 33–47.

25. Guchelaar HJ, Vermes A, Meerwaldt JH (1997). Radiation-induced xerostomia: pathophysiology, clinical course and supportive treatment. *Support Care Cancer* **5**: 281–8.

26. Chambers MS (1997). Xerostomia and its role in mucositis: complications and management. *Support Care Cancer* **5**: 149.

27. Brizel DM, Wasserman TH, Henke M, Strnad V, Rudat V, Monnier A *et al.* (2000). Phase III randomized trial of amifostine as a radioprotector in head and neck cancer. *J Clin Oncol* **18**: 3339–45.

28. Valdez IH, Wolff A, Atkinson JC, Macynski AA, Fox PC (1993). Use of pilocarpine during head and neck radiation therapy to reduce xerostomia and salivary dysfunction. *Cancer* **71**: 1848–51.

29. Rode M, Smid L, Budihna M, Soba E, Rode M, Gaspersic D (1999). The effect of pilocarpine and biperiden on salivary secretion during and after radiotherapy in head and neck cancer patients. *Int J Radiat Oncol Biol Phys* **45**: 373–8.

30. Davies AN (1997). The management of xerostomia: a review. *Eur J Cancer Care* **6**: 209–14.

31. Johnson JT, Ferretti GA, Nethery WJ, Valdez IH, Fox PC, Ng D *et al.* (1993). Oral pilocarpine for post-irradiation xerostomia in patients with head and neck cancer. *New Engl J Med* **329**: 390–5.

32. LeVeque FG, Montgomery M, Potter D, Zimmer MB, Rieke JW, Steiger BW *et al.* (1993). A multicentre, randomized, double-blind, placebo-controlled, dose-titration study of oral pilocarpine for treatment of radiation-induced xerostomia in head and neck cancer patients. *J Clin Oncol* **11**: 1124–31.

33. Johnstone PA, Niemtzow RC, Riffenburgh RH (2002). Acupuncture for xerostomia. *Cancer* **94**: 1151–6.

34. Davies AN, Singer J (1994). A comparison of artificial saliva and pilocarpine in radiation-induced xerostomia. *J Laryngol Otol* **108**: 663–5.

35. Store G, Boysen M (2000). Mandibular osteoradionecrosis: clinical behaviour and diagnostic aspects. *Clinical Otolaryngol* **25**: 378–84.

36. Jereczek-Fossa BA, Orecchia R (2002). Radiotherapy-induced mandibular bone complications. *Cancer Treat Rev* **28**: 65–74.

37. Marx RE (1983). Osteoradionecrosis: a new concept of its pathophysiology. *J Oral Maxillofac Surg* **41**: 283–8.

38. Feldmeier JJ, Hampson NB (2002). A systematic review of the literature reporting the application of hyperbaric oxygen prevention and treatment of delayed radiation injuries: an evidence based approach. *Undersea Hyperb Med* **29**: 4–30.

39. Notani K, Yamazaki Y, Kitada H, Sakakibara N, Fukuda H, Omori K *et al.* (2003). Management of mandibular osteoradionecrosis corresponding to the severity of osteoradionecrosis and the method of radiotherapy. *Head Neck* **25**: 181–6.

40. Chang DW, Oh HK, Robb GL, Miller MJ (2001). Management of advanced mandibular osteoradionecrosis with free flap reconstruction. *Head Neck* **23**: 830–5.

41. Greenberg MS, Cohen SG, McKitrick JC, Cassileth PA (1982). The oral flora as a source of septicemia in patients with acute leukemia. *Oral Surg Oral Med Oral Pathol* **53**: 32–6.

42. Bergmann OJ (1988). Oral infections and septicemia in immunocompromised patients with hematologic malignancies. *J Clin Microbiol* **26**: 2105–9.

Useful websites

National Cancer Institute
http://www.cancer.gov
Cochrane Collaboration
http://www.cochrane.org

Chapter 16

HIV infection/AIDS

Louis DePaola and Arley Silva

Introduction

Oral problems are common in patients with human immunodeficiency virus (HIV) infection/acquired immune deficiency syndrome (AIDS).[1] The presence of oral problems may indicate the presence of HIV infection, the development of AIDS, the progression of HIV infection/AIDS, the failure of antiretroviral therapy, and/or the failure of antimicrobial (prophylactic) therapy.[2]

Generic issues
Background

On 5 June 1981, the Centers for Disease Control and Prevention in the United States of America reported an unusual cluster of *Pneumocystis carinii* pneumonia and other opportunistic infections in five homosexual men.[3] This was the first report of AIDS. By the end of the year 2002, the HIV/AIDS pandemic had infected an estimated 42 million people, with 10 new cases occurring every minute of every day.[4] Figure 16.1 gives a brief history of the first 20 years of the HIV infection/AIDS pandemic.[5–9]

HIV reproduces at a very high rate and in the process of reproduction, HIV kills T-4 helper lymphocytes, also referred to as CD4 lymphocytes, leading to a dramatic decline of immune function.[10] The deterioration of immune function allows for the development of a myriad of opportunistic infections, and also the development of certain malignancies.

Controlling viral replication through the use of highly active antiretroviral therapy (HAART) has markedly reduced the morbidity and mortality from HIV infection.[8,9] HAART regimens vary, but usually consist of at least three drugs, and usually consist of two nucleoside reverse transcriptase inhibitors with either a non-nucleoside reverse transcriptase or a protease inhibitor.[11]

However many patients fail to achieve desired levels of viral suppression because of non-compliance, inability to tolerate antiviral agents, development of viral resistance, or a combination of these factors. Therefore, opportunistic infections and malignancies are still encountered in HIV/AIDS patients, although most are seen with profound

---

1981: Center for Disease Control and Prevention (United States of America) report first cases of AIDS[3]

1983: HIV organism identified[6,7]

1986: First nucleoside reverse transcriptase inhibitor approved for use in USA (zidovudine – AZT)

1995: First protease inhibitor approved for use in USA (saquinavir)

1996: First non-nucleoside reverse transcriptase inhibitor approved for use in USA (nevirapine)

1996: First report of use of combination therapy (highly active antiretroviral therapy – HAART)

1998: Studies report that HAART produces significant reductions in morbidity and mortality[8,9]

2002: HIV infection/AIDS pandemic continues[4]
Number of people living with HIV/AIDS – 42 million (70 per cent in Sub-Saharan Africa)
Number of new infections in 2002 – 5 million
Number of deaths in 2002 – 3.1 million

Fig. 16.1 A brief history of the HIV infection/AIDS pandemic.[5]

immunosuppression (CD4 count <200 cells/mm^3). Appropriate antimicrobial prophylaxis is frequently instituted at this CD4 count.[12]

HAART has evolved into the standard treatment for HIV infection in developed countries.[13] However, in many parts of the world, HAART, or indeed any antiretroviral therapy, is not freely available. Indeed, in many parts of the world, basic supportive therapy is not freely available. Hence, HIV infection/AIDS continues to cause significant morbidity, and significant mortality, throughout the world.[4]

Epidemiology

The reported prevalence of oral lesions in patients with HIV infection varies from 13–99 per cent.[1] There are several explanations for this disparity, including differing populations studied, and differing methodology employed.[1,14]

The types of oral lesion seen varies according to age, gender, mechanism of infection and geographical area.[1] For example, Kaposi's sarcoma is uncommon in children, is more common in male patients, and more common in patients infected as a result of homosexual (male) intercourse.[1]

Aetiology

It has been shown that the prevalence of oral manifestations is significantly related to CD4 cell counts of less than 200 cells/mm^3, and viral loads of greater than 3000 copies/ml.[15] These correlations suggest that oral lesions may be helpful tools for identifying the progression of HIV disease.

Clinical features

A variety of different oral problems are seen in patients with HIV infection/AIDS. Table 16.1 shows a classification of oral problems in infected adults,[16] whilst Table 16.2 shows a classification of orofacial problems in infected children.[17]

There has been a significant decrease in the prevalence of oral lesions in patients on HAART compared with patients not on therapy.[15,18–20] The observation that the prevalence of oral lesions decreases significantly with the administration of HAART suggests that oral lesions can be used as an adjunct clinical marker to monitor the efficacy of antiretroviral therapy.

While the incidence of most opportunistic infections has decreased with HAART, paradoxically the incidence of oral human papillomavirus (HPV) infection has significantly increased (Fig. 16.2).[21,22] Little information is available regarding a possible mechanism for the observed impact of antiretroviral therapy on HPV-associated oral lesions. It has been reported that the occurrence of salivary-gland disease has also increased since the introduction of HAART.[18,21]

Table 16.1 Consensus classification of oral lesions associated with adult HIV infection[16]

Group 1: Lesions strongly associated with HIV infection
Candidiasis ◆ Erythematous ◆ Pseudomembranous
Hairy leukoplakia
Kaposi's sarcoma
Non-Hodgkin's lymphoma
Periodontal disease ◆ Linear gingival erythema ◆ Necrotizing (ulcerative) gingivitis ◆ Necrotizing (ulcerative) periodontitis

Continued

Table 16.1 Consensus classification of oral lesions associated with adult HIV infection[16]—Cont'd

Group 2: Lesions less commonly associated with HIV infection

Bacterial infections
- *Mycobacterium avium-intracellulare*
- *Mycobacterium tuberculosis*

Melanotic hyperpigmentation

Necrotizing (ulcerative) stomatitis

Salivary gland disease
- Dry mouth due to decreased salivary flow rate
- Unilateral or bilateral swelling of major salivary glands

Thrombocytopenic purpura

Ulceration NOS (not otherwise specified)

Viral infections
- Herpes simplex virus
- Human papillomavirus (warty-like) lesions
  – Condyloma acuminatum; Focal epithelial hyperplasia; Verruca vulgaris
- Varicella-zoster virus
  – Herpes zoster; Varicella

Group 3: Lesions seen in HIV infection

Bacterial infections
- *Actinomyces israelii*
- *Escherichia coli*
- *Klebsiella pneumoniae*

Cat-scratch disease

Drug reactions (ulcerative, erythema multiforme, lichenoid, toxic epidermolysis)

Epithelioid (bacillary) angiomatosis

Fungal infection other than candidiasis
- *Cryptococcus neoformans*
- *Geotrichum candidum*
- *Histoplasma capsulatum*
- *Mucoraceae (mucormycosis zygomycosis)*
- *Aspergillus flavus*

Neurologic disturbances
- Facial palsy
- Trigeminal neuralgia

Recurrent aphthous stomatitis

Viral infections
- Cytomegalovirus
- Molluscum contagiosum

Table 16.2 Consensus classification of orofacial lesions associated with paediatric HIV infection[17]

Group 1: Lesions commonly associated with paediatric HIV infection
Candidiasis
◆ Erythematous
◆ Pseudomembranous
◆ Angular cheilitis
Herpes simplex virus infection
Linear gingival erythema
Parotid enlargement
Recurrent aphthous ulcers
◆ Minor
◆ Major
◆ Herpetiform
Group 2: Lesions less commonly associated with paediatric HIV infection
Bacterial infections of oral tissues
Periodontal diseases
◆ Necrotizing (ulcerative) gingivitis
◆ Necrotizing (ulcerative) periodontitis
◆ Necrotizing (ulcerative) stomatitis
Seborrhoeic dermatitis
Viral infections
◆ Cytomegalovirus
◆ Human papillomavirus
◆ Molluscum contagiosum
◆ *Varicella-zoster* virus
– *Herpes zoster; Varicella*
Xerostomia
Group 3: Lesions strongly associated with HIV infection but rare in children
Neoplasms
◆ Kaposi's sarcoma and non-Hodgkin's lymphoma
Oral hairy leukoplakia
Tuberculosis-related ulcers

Management

Oral hygiene

Oral hygiene is an important aspect of the care of patients with HIV infection/AIDS. Studies suggest that intensive oral hygiene regimens improve oral health, oral function and quality of life.[23]

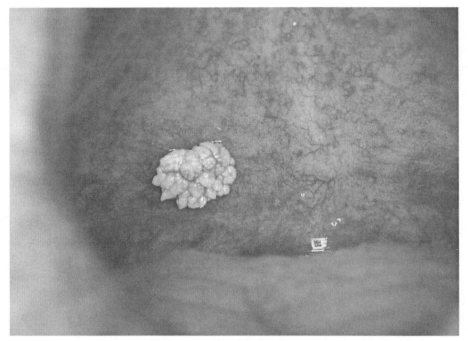

Fig. 16.2 Oral wart. Courtesy of J Eveson. (See also Plate 34 at the centre of this book.)

Dental treatment

The provision of dental care to patients with HIV infection/AIDS can be challenging. The dentistry in itself tends to be very straightforward. However, the dental care is complicated by the presence of HIV infection, the presence of co-morbidity, and the problems associated with antiretroviral therapy (side-effects, drug interactions).

Patients with HIV/AIDS are at increased risk of bleeding/infection following dental treatment. It is essential that patients are fully assessed prior to dental treatment, and that there is close liaison between the dental team and the medical team.[10,24] The assessment should include a complete blood count, together with a differential white cell count.

Antibiotic prophylaxis should be prescribed for individuals who are severely neutropenic (neutrophil count <1000 cells/mm^3), and elective dental procedures should generally be deferred in patients with a neutrophil count <500 cells/mm^3 and/or a platelet count <50,000 cells/mm^3.[10,24] Profoundly neutropenic and thrombocytopenic individuals may receive urgent care as indicated, but hospitalization may be required.

Infection control issues

The risk of acquiring HIV infection from an occupational exposure is real for both medical and dental providers. The transmission rate has been estimated to be ~ 0.3 per cent after a percutaneous injury, and ~ 0.09 per cent after a mucous membrane exposure.[25] As of December 2002, the Centers for Disease Control and Prevention had confirmed 57 cases of HIV seroconversion resulting from occupational exposure amongst American healthcare workers.[26] Several factors play a role in the transmission of HIV after an occupational exposure. Increased risk is associated with exposure to larger quantities of blood, deeper injuries, and a higher titre of HIV in donor blood.[27]

Prevention of occupational exposure is of primary importance. Standard infection control precautions include:

- Hand washing prior to patient contact. Washing hands between patients.
- Routine use of gloves, during procedures likely to involve contact with blood, or other body fluids. Changing gloves between patients.
- Routine use of surgical masks and eye protection, during procedures likely to generate splashes of blood, or other body fluids.
- Careful handling/disposal of contaminated sharps and other equipment.
- Careful handling/disposal of contaminated laundry and other items.

Healthcare personnel should assume that the blood and other body fluids from all patients are potentially infectious.

Post-exposure prophylaxis has been shown to reduce occupational transmission of HIV by as much as 79 per cent.[25] Each and every exposure should be evaluated by a health professional knowledgeable about occupational transmission, and prophylaxis should be instituted, when indicated, as soon as possible.

Specific problems
Oral infections
Oral candidosis

Oral candidosis is the most common oral manifestation of HIV infection, with reported prevalences of up to 94 per cent.[1] There has been a significant decrease in the prevalence of this condition following the introduction of HAART. In most cases, the infection is due to *Candida albicans*. However, other species have been increasingly isolated from HIV patients (e.g. *C. glabrata, C. dubliniensis*).[28]

The clinical features of oral candidosis in HIV patients are similar to those in other patient groups. However, the disease is often more extensive/severe in HIV patients. The most common subtypes are pseudomembranous candidosis, and erythematous candidosis.[28,29] Nevertheless, other subtypes may also occur in patients with HIV infection (e.g. angular cheilitis).

The management of oral candidosis in HIV patients is similar to that in other patient groups. However, oral candidosis is often more difficult to eradicate, and more likely to recur, in HIV patients.[29] Antifungal drug resistance, particularly azole resistance, has been reported to be a particular problem in this group of patients.[30]

Oral candidosis is discussed in detail in Chapter 6.

Oral hairy leukoplakia

Oral hairy leukoplakia is a relatively common oral lesion in HIV patients. The prevalence of oral hairy leukoplakia is influenced by a number of factors. Thus, oral hairy leukoplakia is more common in adults, in males, and in patients infected as a result of homosexual (male) sexual transmission.[1] Oral hairy leukoplakia appears to be related to infection with the Epstein–Barr virus.[28]

Oral hairy leukoplakia usually affects the lateral borders of the tongue, and usually presents as a white, elevated, 'corrugated' lesion (Fig. 16.3).[28,29] However, it can affect other areas (e.g. buccal mucosa), and it can present in other forms (e.g. flat lesions).[31] Oral hairy leukoplakia is usually asymptomatic.

Treatment is generally not indicated/required for oral hairy leukoplakia. However, treatments that have been reported to be effective include local excision, aciclovir

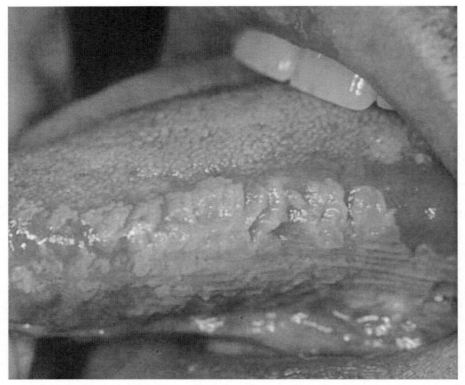

Fig. 16.3 Oral hairy leukoplakia. Courtesy of Dr Valli Meeks. (See also Plate 35 at the centre of this book.)

(intensive courses), podophyllum and tretinoin.[28,31] It should be noted that lesions often improve after the introduction of HAART.[32]

HIV-related periodontal disease

HIV-related periodontal disease has been divided into three main types:[29]

1. Linear gingival erythema ('HIV-associated gingivitis', 'red band gingivitis')
2. Necrotizing ulcerative gingivitis
3. Necrotizing ulcerative periodontitis.

HIV-related periodontal disease is associated with the same bacteria that cause conventional periodontal disease. However, HIV-related periodontal disease is also associated with other 'unusual' bacteria, and with *Candida* species.[29] Other predisposing factors include increasing age, poor oral hygiene and smoking.[29]

Periodontal disease is discussed in detail in Chapter 7.

• Linear gingival erythema

Linear gingival erythema is characterized by a thin, erythematous band along the gingival margin (Fig. 16.4).[28,29] In addition, there may be punctate, or diffuse, erythema of the adjacent gingiva. Patients may complain of bleeding. Linear gingival erythema may progress to necrotizing ulcerative gingivitis (see below).

The management of linear gingival erythema involves good oral hygiene, and dental plaque control measures (e.g. chlorhexidine mouthwashes). Other forms of conventional periodontal treatment may also be required (see Chapter 7).

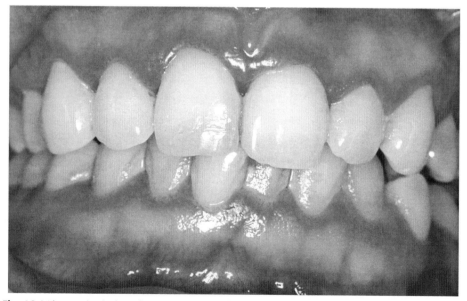

Fig. 16.4 Linear gingival erythema. Courtesy of J Eveson. (See also Plate 36 at the centre of this book.)

- ### Necrotizing ulcerative gingivitis

Necrotizing ulcerative gingivitis may present either acutely, or subacutely: the symptoms include pain, bleeding and halitosis; the signs include necrosis, ulceration and sloughing of the gingival margin/interdental papillae (Fig. 7.5).[29] Necrotizing ulcerative gingivitis may progress to necrotizing stomatitis (i.e. involvement of the oral mucosa).

Initially, treatment consists of local hydrogen peroxide, plus systemic metronidazole. Subsequently, patients require conventional periodontal treatment (i.e. chemical plaque control, scaling, root planing).[29]

- ### Necrotizing ulcerative periodontitis

Necrotizing ulcerative periodontitis is characterized by necrosis/ulceration of the gingiva, together with destruction of the periodontal ligament and alveolar bone (Fig. 16.5).[28,29] Patients may complain of pain (deep-seated), loose teeth, bleeding and halitosis. Necrotizing ulcerative periodontitis may progress to necrotizing ulcerative stomatitis (see above).

The management of necrotizing ulcerative periodontitis involves debridement of necrotic tissue, topical antimicrobial agents (chlorhexidine, povidone iodine), systemic antibiotics (metronidazole, tetracycline), and other forms of conventional periodontal treatment.

Oral neoplasms

Kaposi's sarcoma (epidemic Kaposi's sarcoma)

Kaposi's sarcoma is the most common malignancy in patients with HIV infection, with a reported prevalence of oral involvement of up to 38 per cent.[1] However, as discussed

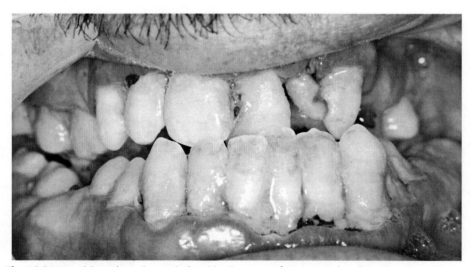

Fig. 16.5 Necrotizing ulcerative periodontitis. Courtesy of Dr Jane Luker. (See also Plate 37 at the centre of this book.)

above, the prevalence of this condition has decreased since the introduction of HAART. Kaposi's sarcoma is more common in adults, in males, and in patients infected as a result of homosexual (male) sexual transmission.[1] It is associated with infection with human herpes virus 8, which is also known as Kaposi's sarcoma-associated herpes virus.[33]

Kaposi's sarcoma often affects the skin, and can affect almost any other part of the body. Oral lesions occur in ~ 35 per cent patients.[34] Oral lesions are usually sited on the gingivae and palate. Lesions can occur in isolation or in groups, may vary in colour from red to purple, may vary (progress) in size from millimetres to centimetres, and may vary (progress) in form from macules to nodules (Fig. 16.6). The lesions may be asymptomatic, or may cause a variety of local symptoms (e.g. oral discomfort, bleeding, difficulty eating, difficulty speaking).[31,34]

There is no curative treatment for Kaposi's sarcoma. The decision to treat/how to treat Kaposi's sarcoma depends on a number of factors, including the patient's general condition, the extent of the disease, the symptomatology of the lesions and the potential side-effects of the treatment. Local treatments include excision, cryotherapy, laser therapy, radiotherapy and intralesional chemotherapy.[33,34] Systemic treatments include single agent chemotherapy, combination chemotherapy, immunotherapy (α interferon), and anti-angiogenesis drugs (thalidomide).[33,34] It should be noted that lesions often improve after the introduction of HAART.[35]

Non-Hodgkin's lymphoma (AIDS-related non-Hodgkin's lymphoma)

Non-Hodgkin's lymphoma (NHL) is a relatively common malignancy in patients with HIV infection with a reported prevalence of oral involvement of up to 5 per cent.[1]

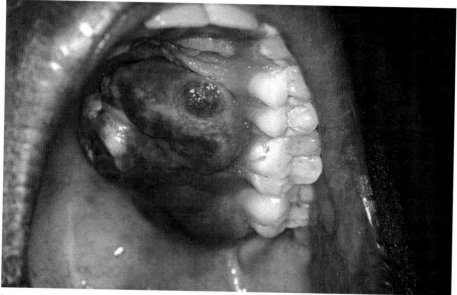

Fig. 16.6 Kaposi's sarcoma. Courtesy of A Davies. (See also Plate 38 at the centre of this book.)

The prevalence of this condition has also decreased somewhat since the introduction of HAART.[33] AIDS-related lymphomas are associated with infection with both Epstein–Barr virus, and also human herpes virus 8.[33] In general, AIDS-related lymphomas are high-grade, B-cell lymphomas.[34]

At presentation, most patients have widespread disease (nodal/extranodal involvement). Moreover, most patients have associated 'B' symptoms, i.e. weight loss, fever, and sweats. Oral lesions can be sited throughout the oral cavity, including the gingivae, palate, buccal mucosae, tongue and tonsils. Lesions may vary in form from ulcers to nodules.[31,34]

The decision to treat/how to treat NHL depends on a number of factors, including the patient's general condition, the extent of the disease and the potential side-effects of the treatment. Local treatment invariably involves radiotherapy. Systemic treatment invariably involves combination chemotherapy. In general, 'good risk' patients are treated with conventional regimens, whilst 'poor risk' patients are treated with modified/low dose regimens.[33,34]

References

1. Patton LL, Phelan JA, Ramos-Gomez FJ, Nittayananta W, Shiboski CH, Mbuguye TL (2002). Prevalence and classification of HIV-associated oral lesions. *Oral Dis* **8** Suppl 2: 98–109.

2. Greenspan JS, Greenspan D (2002). The epidemiology of the oral lesions of HIV infection in the developed world. *Oral Dis* **8** Suppl 2: 34–9.

3. Anonymous (1981). *Pneumocystis* pneumonia – Los Angeles. *MMWR Morb Mortal Wkly Rep* **30**: 250–2.

4. Joint United Nations Programme on HIV/AIDS (UNAIDS) and World Health Organization (WHO) (2002). *AIDS epidemic update: December 2002*. Geneva: UNAIDS and WHO.

5. Bartlett JG (2001). HIV: twenty years in review. *Hopkins HIV Rep* **13**: 8–9.

6. Gallo RC, Sarin PS, Gelmann EP, Robert-Guroff M, Richardson E, Kalyanaraman VS *et al.* (1983). Isolation of human T-cell leukemia virus in acquired immune deficiency syndrome (AIDS). *Science* **220**: 865–7.

7. Barre-Sinoussi F, Chermann JC, Rey F, Nugeyre MT, Chamaret S, Gruest J *et al.* (1983). Isolation of a T-lymphotropic retrovirus from a patient at risk for acquired immune deficiency syndrome (AIDS). *Science* **220**: 868–71.

8. Palella FJ, Delaney KM, Moorman AC, Loveless MO, Fuhrer J, Satten GA *et al.* (1998). Declining morbidity and mortality among patients with advanced human immunodeficiency virus infection. *N Engl J Med* **338**: 853–60.

9. Mocroft A, Vella S, Benfield TL, Chiesi A, Miller V, Gargalianos P *et al.* (1998). Changing patterns of mortality across Europe in patients infected with HIV-1. EuroSIDA Study Group. *Lancet* **352**: 1725–30.

10. Bartlett JG, Gallant JE (2003). *Medical Management of HIV Infection*. Baltimore: John Hopkins University.

11. Luzzi GA, Peto TE, Weiss RA, Conlon CP (2003). HIV and AIDS. In DA Warrell, TM Cox, JD Firth, EJ Benz Jr (ed.) *Oxford Textbook of Medicine*, 4th edn, p. 431. Oxford: Oxford University Press.

12. Kaplan JE, Masur H, Holmes KK (2002). USPHS. Infectious Diseases Society of America. Guidelines for preventing opportunistic infections among HIV-infected persons – 2002. Recommendations of the U.S. Public Health Service and the Infectious Diseases Society of America. *MMWR Recomm Rep* **51** (RR-8): 1–52.

13. Department of Health and Human Services (DHHS) (2003). *Guidelines for the use of Antiretroviral Agents in HIV-1-infected Adults and Adolescents*. Washington DC: DHSS.

14. Holmes HK, Stephen LX (2002). Oral lesions of HIV infection in developing countries. *Oral Dis* **8**, Suppl 2: 40–3.

15. Tappuni AR, Fleming GJ (2001). The effect of antiretroviral therapy on the prevalence of oral manifestations in HIV-infected patients: a UK study. *Oral Surg Oral Med Oral Pathol Oral Radiol Endod* **92**: 623–8.

16. Anonymous (1993). Classification and diagnostic criteria for oral lesions in HIV infection. EC- Clearinghouse on Oral Problems Related to HIV Infection and WHO Collaborating Centre on Oral Manifestations of the Immunodeficiency Virus. *J Oral Pathol Med* **22**: 289–91.

17. Ramos-Gomez FJ, Flaitz C, Catapano P, Murray P, Milnes AR, Dorenbaum A (1999). Classification, diagnostic criteria, and treatment recommendations for orofacial manifestations in HIV-infected pediatric patients. Collaborative Workgroup on Oral Manifestations of Pediatric HIV Infection. *J Clin Pediatr Dent* **23**: 85–96.

18. Patton LL, McKaig R, Strauss R, Rogers D, Eron JJ Jr, Hill C (2000). Changing prevalence of oral manifestations of human immunodeficiency virus in the era of protease inhibitor therapy. *Oral Surg Oral Med Oral Pathol Oral Radiol Endod* **89**: 299–304.

19. Schmidt-Westhausen AM, Priepke F, Bergmann FJ, Reichart PA (2000). Decline in the rate of oral opportunistic infections following introduction of highly active antiretroviral therapy. *J Oral Pathol Med* **29**: 336–41.

20. Eyeson JD, Tenant-Flowers M, Cooper DJ, Johnson NW, Warnakulasuriya KA (2002). Oral manifestations of an HIV positive cohort in the era of highly active anti-retroviral therapy (HAART) in South London. *J Oral Pathol Med* **31**: 169–74.

21. Greenspan D, Canchola AJ, MacPhail LA, Cheikh B, Greenspan JS (2001). Effect of highly active antiretroviral therapy on the frequency of oral warts. *Lancet* **357**: 1411–12.

22. King MD, Reznik DA, O'Daniels CM, Larsen NM, Osterholt D, Blumberg HM (2002). Human papillomavirus-associated oral warts among human immunodeficiency virus-seropositive patients in the era of highly active antiretroviral therapy: an emerging infection. *Clin Infect Dis* **34**: 641–8.

23. Brown JB, Rosenstein D, Mullooly J, O'Keefe Rosetti M, Robinson S, Chiodo G (2002). Impact of intensified dental care on outcomes in human immunodeficiency virus infection. *AIDS Patient Care STDS* **16**: 479–86.

24. Patton LL, Glick M (2001). *Clinician's Guide to HIV-infected Patients*, 3rd edn. Baltimore: The American Academy of Oral Medicine.

25. U.S. Public Health Service (2001). Updated U.S. Public Health Service guidelines for the management of occupational exposures to HBV, HCV, and HIV and recommendations for postexposure prophylaxis. *MMWR Recomm Rep* **50** (RR-11): 1–52.

26. Centers for Disease Control and Prevention (CDC) (2002). *Preventing occupational HIV transmission to healthcare personnel: February 2002*. Atlanta: CDC.

27. Cardo DM, Culver DH, Ciesielski CA, Srivastava PU, Marcus R, Abiteboul D *et al.* (1997). A case-control study of HIV seroconversion in health care workers after percutaneous exposure. Centers for Disease Control and Prevention Needlestick Surveillance Group. *N Engl J Med* **337**: 1485–90.

28. Casiglia JW, Woo S (2000). Oral manifestations of HIV infection. *Clin Dermatol* **18**: 541–51.

29. Laskaris G (2000). Oral manifestations of HIV disease. *Clin Dermatol* **18**: 447–55.

30. Denning DW, Baily GG, Hood SV (1997). Azole resistance in *Candida*. *Eur J Clin Microbiol Infect Dis* **16**: 261–80.

31. Greenspan JS, Greenspan D (1997). Oral disease in human immunodeficiency infection. In VT DeVita Jr, S Hellman, SA Rosenberg (ed.) *AIDS. Etiology, Diagnosis, Treatment and Prevention*, 4th edn. Philadelphia: Lippincott-Raven Publishers.

32. Albrecht H, Stellbrink H-J, Brewster D, Greten H (1994). Resolution of oral hairy leukoplakia. *AIDS* **8**: 1014–16.

33. Scadden DT (2003). AIDS-related malignancies. *Annu Rev Med* **54**: 285–303.

34. Tirelli U, Spina M, Carbone A, Monfardini S (2002). Neoplastic complications of AIDS. In RL Souhami, I Tannock, P Hohenberger, J-C Horiot. *Oxford Textbook of Oncology*, 2nd edn. Oxford: Oxford University Press.

35. Tavio M, Nasti G, Spina M, Errante D, Vaccher E, Tirelli U (1998). Highly active antiretroviral therapy in HIV-related Kaposi's sarcoma. *Ann Oncol* **9**: 923.

Useful websites

Joint United Nations Programme on HIV/AIDS
http://www.unaids.org
Centers for Disease Control and Prevention
http://www.cdc.gov
AIDSinfo (United States Department of Health and Human Services)
http://www.aidsinfo.nih.gov
HIVdent
http://www.hivdent.org

Chapter 17

Chronic neurological diseases

Janice Fiske

Introduction

Oral problems are common in patients with advanced chronic neurological diseases.[1] Moreover, oral problems may have a significant impact on the quality of life of this group of patients. The first part of the chapter will consider generic issues for patients with advanced chronic neurological diseases, whilst the second part of the chapter will consider specific issues for patients with Alzheimer's disease, Parkinson's disease, multiple sclerosis, and motor neurone disease.

Generic issues
Oral assessment/planning

Every patient with advanced chronic neurological disease should have an oral assessment performed, and an oral plan formulated. The oral assessment provides a mechanism for opportunistic identification of people who require help with daily oral hygiene, people who have oral problems, and people who have dental problems (and who require attention from the dental team). The oral assessment should be repeated at regular intervals, and the oral plan revised as necessary.

Figure 17.1 shows an oral assessment tool that can be used in patients with chronic neurological diseases. The tool in the figure has been adapted from the tool in the British Society for Disability and Oral Health guidelines.[2]

Oral problems may present as behavioural changes in patients with cognitive impairment and/or communication problems. Changes in behaviour which can be indicative of an oral problem include:

- Pulling at the face
- Refusal to eat, e.g. cold food
- Non-wearing of dentures
- Increased drooling
- Increased vocalization, e.g. shouting
- Increased restlessness
- Disturbed sleep

Name of client: _____

Date of birth: _____

Hospital number: _____

1. Does the client have natural teeth?

No ☐ Yes ☐ Uncertain ☐

2. Does the client wear dentures?

No ☐ Yes ☐ Uncertain ☐

a) If Yes, specify whether dentures worn are

Upper ☐ Lower ☐

b) If Yes, are the dentures labelled?

No ☐ Yes ☐

c) If Yes, are the dentures in obvious need of repair?

No ☐ Yes ☐

3. Does the client have any problems?

No ☐ Yes ☐ Uncertain ☐

e.g. pain, difficulty eating, decayed teeth,

dry mouth, ulcers, halitosis, other, etc.?

a) If Yes, specify whether

Teeth ☐ Gums ☐ Denture ☐ Other ☐

b) If Yes, describe the problem(s) _____
_____

Fig. 17.1 Oral health assessment tool for patients with chronic neurological diseases.

4. Does the client smoke?	No ☐	Yes ☐	Uncertain ☐
5. Is the client on medication with oral side effects, e.g. dry mouth?	No ☐	Yes ☐	Uncertain ☐
6. Does the client need urgent dental treatment?	No ☐	Yes ☐	Uncertain ☐
7. Does the client need to see a member of the dental team?	No ☐	Yes ☐	Uncertain ☐
8. Does the client need help with cleaning their dentures?	No ☐	Yes ☐	Uncertain ☐
9. Does the client need help with cleaning their teeth?	No ☐	Yes ☐	Uncertain ☐
10. The following mouth care is required for this client on a daily basis: a) b) c)			

Fig. 17.1 Cont'd

- Refusal to undertake normal activities of daily living
- Self-injurious behaviour; and
- Aggressive behaviour towards carers.[3]

Oral hygiene

It is important a balance is struck between maintaining independence and maintaining adequate oral hygiene. Initially, the patient may be able to maintain this function with the aid of an adapted toothbrush, or an electric toothbrush (see Fig. 3.1).

Subsequently, however, a carer will need to undertake this function. The carer needs instruction on how to approach this task. The technique will vary depending on the individual concerned. Generally, the easiest method is to have the patient seated on a dining chair, with the carer stood behind them: the patient's head is cradled by one of the carer's arms, and supported against the carer's body. This position provides adequate control of the head, and good vision of the mouth. In certain cases, it may be necessary to have another person to support the head, or to hold the hands (see Chapter 3).

Patients with advanced chronic neurological diseases are at increased risk of aspiration. Maintaining oral hygiene, particularly removing retained food debris, can decrease the risks. Oral hygiene and denture care are discussed in detail in Chapter 3.

Dental treatment

Ideally, dental professionals (dentists, dental hygienists) should be part of the multidisciplinary team caring for patients with chronic neurological diseases. Involvement of the dental team should take the form of routine reviews, routine treatments, as well as 'crisis' management. (Involvement of the dental team should occur at all stages of the disease.) Dental care can be undertaken in the dental surgery, or in the domiciliary setting (see Chapter 4).

In the early stages of the disease most dental treatment care is possible. Key teeth (canines, molars, occluding pairs) should be identified and, if necessary, restored to function. Similarly, dental prostheses (dentures, other prostheses) should be assessed and, if required, altered or replaced. Any treatment should be high quality, and low maintenance. Preventive measures should also be put in place at this stage, such as use of fluoride and/or chlorhexidine mouthwashes. As the disease progresses, the focus of dental treatment should be on maintenance of function. However, preventative measures should be continued. In the late stages of the disease, the focus of dental treatment is on the palliation of symptoms.

Even though the patient may have cognitive impairment and/or communication problems, it is important that they are informed and, whenever possible, involved in the decision-making process. In such circumstances, it is prudent also to involve the family or carers in the decision-making process. However, even when agreement is gained from the family or carers, it is advisable that 'professional consent' is sought in instances where the proposed treatment is irreversible, i.e. two independent healthcare professionals should agree that the proposed treatment is in the best interests of the patient.

Dietary issues

Poor nutrition and weight loss are major concerns in this group of patients. Increased nutrient intake is encouraged by the consumption of: (a) frequent snacks; (b) food enrichment; and (c) food supplements. The long-term consumption of high sugar foodstuffs can have a detrimental effect on oral health (dental caries). The problem is compounded by difficulty swallowing (sugar not swallowed promptly), and/or dry mouth (sugar acids not buffered properly). Rigorous oral hygiene measures can help to prevent such problems.[4] Similarly, strategies to improve dysphagia and/or dry mouth can also be helpful.

Generic oral problems
Dry mouth

Dry mouth is a very common complaint in patients with chronic neurological diseases. The cause of the problem is usually drug treatment. The strategies used to manage dry mouth are discussed in Chapter 9.

Tenacious secretions

Tenacious secretions accumulating in the oropharynx is a relatively common complaint in patients with chronic neurological diseases. The cause of the problem is usually a combination of dry mouth and difficulty swallowing. The strategies used to manage tenacious secretions include treatment of dry mouth, humidification,[5] soda water,[6] fruit juices (dark grape, pineapple)[6] and beta blockers (propranolol 10mg twice daily, metoprolol 25mg twice daily).[7]

Drooling

Drooling is defined as 'abnormal spillage of saliva from the mouth on to the lips, chin and clothing'.[8]

In patients with chronic neurological diseases, drooling is usually related to difficulty in removing saliva from the mouth (secondary to dysphagia), and/or difficulty in retaining saliva within the mouth (secondary to facial weakness). Drooling is usually not related to increased secretion of saliva.

Drooling is associated with a number of physical, psychological, and social problems:[9]

- Physical – maceration perioral skin, secondary infection perioral skin, malodour.
- Psychological – low self-esteem, anxiety, depression.
- Social – clothing issues, laundry issues, social isolation.

Table 17.1 Interventions for the management of drooling in patients with chronic neurological diseases

Intervention		Comment
Non pharmacological methods	Behavioural therapy[11] Intra oral appliances [12]	The aim of this intervention is to increase swallowing The aim of this intervention is to improve mouth closure
Pharmacological methods	Drugs Botulinum toxin A[13]	See Table 15.2
Radiotherapy	Salivary gland radiotherapy[14]	
Surgery	Parasympathetic nerve ablation[15] Salivary gland duct ligation Salivary gland duct relocation Salivary gland excision	Surgery is usually not indicated in palliative care patients
Complementary therapies	Acupuncture[16]	Acupuncture of the tongue has been reported to be effective in children with drooling secondary to neurological problems

A number of strategies have been employed to control drooling.[10] However, some of these options are not appropriate for patients with advanced/end-stage neurological diseases. The strategies that have been used to control drooling in this group of patients are shown in Table 17.1. The choice of treatment depends on a number of factors, including the patient's performance status, the patient's prognosis, the distress caused by the drooling and (particularly) the patient's choice of treatment.

Drugs are the mainstay of treatment in patients with advanced/end stage neurological diseases. The drug regimens that have been reported to control drooling in this group of patients are shown in Table 17.2. Nevertheless, other drug regimens are used to control drooling in clinical practice. The principles of drug use are:

1. Start at a low dose;
2. Titrate the dose in small increments;
3. Titrate the dose upwards if symptoms persist;
4. Titrate the dose downwards if side-effects develop.

It is particularly important not to substitute a relatively benign problem (drooling), for a more malignant problem (dry mouth).

Denture problems

Patients with chronic neurological diseases often have problems wearing/retaining dentures: denture-wearing success depends to a large extent on the functioning

Table 17.2 Drugs used in the management of drooling in patients with chronic neurological diseases

Drug*	Route*	Dose*
Atropine	Oral,[17] sublingual[18]	Oral dose 0.25–0.75mg/24 hr[17] Sublingual dose 0.5mg b.d.[18]
Benzatropine	Oral[17]	Oral dose 1–2mg/24 hr[17]
Hyoscine hydrobromide	Transdermal,[17] nebulized[19]	Transdermal dose 1–2mg/72 hr[17] Nebulized dose 0.8mg b.d. – t.d.s.[19]
Glycopyrronium	PEG tube,[20] nebulized,[21] parenteral[17]	PEG tube dose 0.6–1mg t.d.s.[20] Nebulized dose 0.4mg b.d.[21] Parenteral dose 0.1–0.2mg b.d.[17]
Amitriptyline	Oral[17]	Oral dose 10–150mg/24 hr[17]
Trihexyphenidyl	Oral[17]	Oral dose 6–10mg/24 hr[17]
Clonidine	Oral[17]	Oral dose 0.15–0.3mg/24 hr[17]

*Other drugs, other routes, and other doses are used to manage drooling in patients with chronic neurological diseases.

of the oral musculature, and also on the presence of an adequate amount of saliva. In some individuals the use of a denture fixative will suffice, whilst in other individuals (with poor-fitting dentures) relining or replacement of the denture will be necessary. Some individuals are unable to cope with their dentures in spite of these strategies.

Replacing dentures can be challenging, if not impossible, in patients with chronic neurological diseases. (Individuals do not possess the necessary cooperation.) Furthermore, if the patient is without their denture for any length of time, they can lose their denture-wearing skills.

Denture loss is not unusual in the various care settings (nursing homes, hospitals). It is good practice to mark dentures with the person's name, since this may help them to be reunited, should they become separated. The techniques used to mark dentures are discussed in Chapter 3.

Specific problems
Alzheimer's disease/other dementias[22]

Alzheimer's disease results in cognitive impairment, although physical deterioration also occurs. Both of these factors may impact on the patient's ability to maintain oral hygiene. Indeed, poor oral hygiene (leading to periodontal disease/dental caries) is the predominant oral problem in this group of patients. The condition, and many of the treatments that are used in this condition, may cause xerostomia, which will exacerbate the oral problems.

Table 17.3 Oral problems in patients with Parkinson's disease[24]

Oral problem	Prevalence (%)
Xerostomia	55
Dysphagia	48
Loose dentures	31
Sore gums	23
Ulcers	17
Bleeding gums	12
Burning sensation	10
Loose teeth	8
Sore teeth	5.

Parkinson's disease[23]

The clinical features of Parkinson's disease relate to impaired motor function, although patients may have associated cognitive problems. The motor problems affect the person's ability to maintain oral hygiene. Furthermore, localized motor problems may lead to difficulty opening the mouth, drooling, difficulty chewing, difficulty swallowing and difficulty speaking. Other features include involuntary movements and rigidity of the orofacial musculature. The drugs used to manage the symptoms of Parkinson's disease may cause xerostomia, which may lead to further oral problems. Patients with Parkinson's disease may also have taste disturbance. Table 17.3 shows the prevalence of oral problems in a mixed group of patients with Parkinson's disease.[24] It should be noted that burning mouth appears to be particularly common in patients with Parkinson's disease.[25]

Multiple sclerosis[26]

Multiple sclerosis results in motor problems, sensory problems and cognitive impairment. All of these factors may impact on the patient's ability to maintain oral hygiene. Many of the treatments that are used in this condition may cause xerostomia, which will exacerbate the oral problems. The motor problems may result in a number of symptoms, including drooling, difficulty chewing, difficulty swallowing and difficulty speaking. The incidence of orofacial problems in a mixed group of patients with multiple sclerosis is shown in Table 17.4.[27] It should be noted that trigeminal neuralgia is a characteristic feature of patients with multiple sclerosis.[28]

Motor neurone disease (amyotrophic lateral sclerosis)[17]

The clinical features of motor neurone disease relate to impaired motor function, although patients may have associated cognitive problems. The muscle weakness

Table 17.4 Orofacial problems in patients with multiple sclerosis[27]

Orofacial problem	Incidence (%)
Orofacial paraesthesia	37
Orofacial pain	30
Taste disturbance	23
Difficulty swallowing	22
Orofacial muscle spasm/palsy	17
Difficulty chewing	8

affects the person's ability to maintain oral hygiene. Furthermore, localized muscle weakness may lead to drooling, difficulty chewing, difficulty swallowing, and difficulty speaking. Other features include muscle cramps, and spasticity of the orofacial muscu-lature. (Patients with pseudobulbar disease may develop jaw quivering/jaw clenching in response to noxious stimuli, e.g. anxiety, pain, the cold). The drugs used to manage the symptoms of motor neurone disease may cause xerostomia, which may lead to further oral problems. Patients with motor neurone disease may also develop problems with accumulation of tenacious secretions in the oropharynx.

References

1. Kieser J, Jones G, Borlase G, MacFadyen E (1999). Dental treatment of patients with neurodegenerative disease. *N Z Dent J* **95**: 130–4.
2. British Society for Disability and Oral Health (2000). Guidelines for oral health care for people with a physical disability. Available from URL: http://www.bsdh.org.uk
3. Ettinger RL (2000). Dental management of patients with Alzheimer's disease and other dementias. *Gerodontology* **17**: 8–16.
4. Hyland K, Fiske J, Mathews N (2000). Nutritional and dental health management in Parkinson's disease. *J Community Nurs* **14**: 28–32.
5. Scott A, Foulsum M (2000). Speech and language therapy. In D Oliver, GD Borasio, D Walsh (ed.) *Palliative Care in Amyotrophic Lateral Sclerosis*, p. 121. Oxford: Oxford University Press.
6. Anonymous (2000). *Practical Management of Motor Neurone Disease: speech pathology*, 3rd edn. Caulfield: Bethlehem Hospital Inc.
7. Newall AR, Orser R, Hunt M (1996). The control of oral secretions in bulbar ALS/MND. *J Neurol Sci* **139** Suppl: 43–4.
8. Brodsky L (1993). Drooling in children. In JC Arvedson and L Brodsky (ed.) *Pediatric Swallowing and Feeding: assessment and management*. San Diego, CA: Singular Publishing Group.
9. Kilpatrick NM, Johnson H, Reddihough D (2000). Sialorrhea: a multidisciplinary approach to the management of drooling children. *Journal of Disability and Oral Health* **1**: 3–9.
10. Hussein I, Kershaw AE, Tahmassebi JF, Fayle SA (1998). The management of drooling in children and patients with mental and physical disabilities: a literature review. *Int J Paediatr Dent* **8**: 3–11.
11. Marks L, Turner K, O'Sullivan J, Deighton B, Lees A (2001). Drooling in Parkinson's disease: a novel speech and language therapy intervention. *Int J Lang Commun Disord* **36**: 282–7.

12. Moulding MB, Koroluk LD (1991). An intraoral prosthesis to control drooling in a patient with amyotrophic lateral sclerosis. *Spec Care Dentist* **11**: 200–2.

13. Porta M, Gamba M, Bertacchi G, Vaj P (2001). Treatment of sialorrhoea with ultrasound guided botulinum toxin type A injection in patients with neurological disorders. *J Neurol Neurosurg Psychiatry* **70**: 538–40.

14. Borg M, Hirst F (1998). The role of radiation therapy in the management of sialorrhea. *Int J Radiat Oncol Biol Phys* **41**: 1113–19.

15. Goode RL, Smith RA (1970). The surgical management of sialorrhea. *Laryngoscope* **80**: 1078–89.

16. Wong V, Sun JG, Wong W (2001). Traditional Chinese medicine (tongue acupuncture) in children with drooling problems. *Pediatr Neurol* **25**: 47–54.

17. Borasio GD, Oliver D (2000). The control of other symptoms. In D Oliver, GD Borasio, D Walsh (ed.) *Palliative Care in Amyotrophic Lateral Sclerosis*, p. 75. Oxford: Oxford University Press.

18. Hyson HC, Johnson AM, Jog MS (2002). Sublingual atropine for sialorrhea secondary to parkinsonism: a pilot study. *Mov Disord* **6**: 1318–20.

19. Zeppetella G (1999). Nebulized scopolamine in the management of oral dribbling: three case reports. *J Pain Symptom Manage* **17**: 293–5.

20. Lucas V (1998). Use of enteral glycopyrollate in the management of drooling. *Palliat Med* **12**: 207–8.

21. Strutt R, Fardell B, Chye R (2002). Nebulized glycopyrrolate for drooling in a motor neuron patient. *J Pain Symptom Manage* **23**: 2–3.

22. Ghezzi EM, Ship JA (2000). Dementia and oral health. *Oral Surg Oral Med Oral Pathol Oral Radiol Endod* **89**: 2–5.

23. Fiske J, Hyland K (2000). Parkinson's disease and oral care. *Dent Update* **27**: 58–65.

24. Clifford T, Finnerty J (1995). The dental awareness and needs of a Parkinson's disease population. *Gerodontology* **12**: 99–103.

25. Clifford TJ, Warsi MJ, Burnett CA, Lamey PJ (1998). Burning mouth in Parkinson's disease sufferers. *Gerodontology* **15**: 73–8.

26. Fiske J, Griffiths J, Thompson S (2002). Multiple sclerosis and oral care. *Dent Update* **29**: 273–83.

27. Fabiano JA (1983). Orofacial involvement in multiple sclerosis. *Spec Care Dent* **3**: 61–4.

28. Friedlander AH, Zeff S (1974). Atypical trigeminal neuralgia in patients with multiple sclerosis. *J Oral Surg* **32**: 301–3.

Useful websites

British Society for Disability and Oral Health
http://www.bsdh.org.uk

Chapter 18

Paediatric problems

Richard Hain, Graham Roberts and Victoria Lucas

Introduction

Although there are many common features, there are also some major differences between paediatric and adult palliative care.[1]

The Association for Children with Life-threatening or Terminal Conditions and their Families/The Royal College of Paediatrics and Child Health (United Kingdom) definition of paediatric palliative care is shown in Fig. 18.1, whilst their categorization of 'life-limiting conditions' is shown in Fig. 18.2.[1] It can be seen that many children receiving palliative care will have non-malignant disease, and will have long-term requirements.

It is axiomatic among those looking after them that 'children are not small adults'. This principle can perhaps be overstated: a child who is unconscious and ventilated can, if seen in isolation from his family and home, be considered with some legitimacy to be little different from a scaled down adult. But there the similarities end. The child's understanding of disease, his concepts of death, his social functioning – all dimensions other than the purely physical, in fact – are profoundly different from those of an adult.

The aim of this chapter is to review the oral problems associated with the more common paediatric life-limiting conditions.

Oral problems of sick children

In general terms, the oral problems of sick children are related to the oral problems that occur within the general paediatric population, i.e. dental caries, gingivitis, and periodontitis (and their complications).

The increased frequency of dental caries is related to a number of factors, including poor oral hygiene (secondary to disability), poor diet (high sugar content), dry mouth (secondary to medication) and use of paediatric medication (high sugar content). It should be noted that children with chronic diseases appear to receive more radical interventional treatment as compared to children without such diseases, i.e. more extractions and less restorations.[2] Dental caries is discussed in detail in Chapter 7.

In addition, sick children may develop a variety of other oral problems. The oral problems may be related to a direct effect of the underlying disease, an indirect effect of the underlying disease, and/or an effect of the treatment for the disease (see below).

Palliative care for children and young people with life-limiting conditions is an active and total approach to care, embracing physical, emotional, social and spiritual elements. It focuses on enhancement of quality of life for the child and support for the family and includes the management of distressing symptoms, provision of respite and care through death and bereavement.

Fig. 18.1 Definition of paediatric palliative care.[1]

- Life-threatening conditions for which curative treatment may be feasible but can fail (e.g. cancer).

- Conditions where premature death is inevitable, where there may be long periods of intensive treatment aimed at prolonging life and allowing participation in normal activities (e.g. cystic fibrosis).

- Progressive conditions without curative treatment options, where treatment is exclusively palliative and may commonly extend over many years (e.g. Duchenne muscular dystrophy).

- Irreversible but non-progressive conditions causing severe disability leading to susceptibility to health complications and likelihood of premature death (e.g. severe cerebral palsy).

Fig. 18.2 Categories of life-limiting paediatric conditions.[1]

Oral care of sick children

Children need to be cared for by those trained in, and accustomed to, working with them. The management of oral symptoms is often complex and multidimensional. For it to be done well requires the skills not only of paediatricians and children's nursing staff, but also of paediatric dentists, dental hygienists, dieticians, speech and language therapists and many others.

The principles of management of oral problems in children are essentially the same as those in adults. Nevertheless, the care given will need to be modified according to the age, diagnosis and ability/disability of the child. In particular, the dose of medication needs to be based on the age, body weight, or body surface area of the child.

Table 18.1 Prevalence of certain oral symptoms amongst paediatric oncology patients[4]

Problem	Overall prevalence %	Leukaemia group %	Lymphoma group %	Solid tumour group %	CNS tumour group %
Dry mouth	31	22	12	41	56
Taste disturbance	17	9	8	28	12
Mouth sores	14	9	15	20	6
Difficulty swallowing	13	3	4	19	11

Doses of medications for children can be found in paediatric formularies, such as the one produced by the Royal College of Paediatrics and Child Health/Neonatal and Paediatric Pharmacists Group (United Kingdom).[3]

Malignant disease

There is relatively little data on the prevalence of oral problems in children with malignant disease, particularly children with advanced malignant disease. Table 18.1 shows the reported prevalence of some oral problems in a mixed group of children with malignant disease.[4]

As discussed above, oral problems may be related to the cancer (directly or indirectly), or to the cancer treatment. Moreover, oral problems may occur at all stages of the cancer journey (at diagnosis, during treatment, during remission, at recurrence). Indeed, oral problems can be seen in the long-term survivors of cancer.[5]

Oral problems cause morbidity per se, but may also lead to secondary physical and psychological problems (see below). Indeed, oral problems can result in a significant deterioration in quality of life. Table 18.2 shows the impact of some oral problems in a mixed group of children with malignant disease.[4]

One of the most common problems is oral discomfort/pain. Broadly speaking, a child will develop a painful or uncomfortable mouth, because the mouth has become

Table 18.2 Characteristics of certain oral symptoms amongst paediatric oncology patients[4]

Problem	Overall prevalence %	Symptomatic patients		
		Intensity – 'moderate' to 'very severe' %	Frequency – 'a lot' to 'almost always' %	Distress – 'quite a bit' to 'very much' %
Dry mouth	31	50	29	24
Taste disturbance	17	77	N/A	30
Mouth sores	14	59	N/A	57
Difficulty swallowing	13	84	56	76

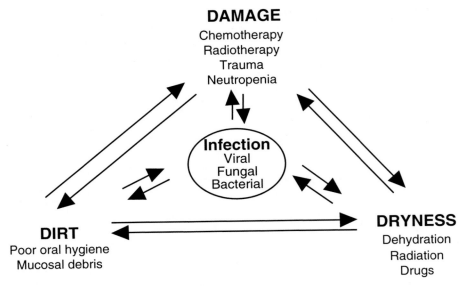

Fig. 18.3 Aetiology of oral discomfort/pain.

damaged, dirty, dry, or infected (Fig. 18.3). Since any one of these problems predisposes to all of the others, it is not unusual to find at any one time all of them coexisting.

Oral discomfort/pain is much more than a physical problem. The child with a sore mouth often chooses not to eat or drink in order to avoid the discomfort. The urge to nourish and sustain one's offspring is a basic one, and the sight of their child refusing food and drink because of pain is one that profoundly affects parents. Their anxiety is quickly recognized by the whole family, who become anxious in their turn. The effect of this apparently simple physical problem therefore has ramifications into every area of the dynamic of the family.

Disease-related problems

As discussed above, oral problems may be related to a direct effect of the malignancy. For example, patients with acute leukaemia may present with gingival enlargement as a result of tumour infiltration.[6] In addition, oral problems may be related to an indirect effect of the malignancy. For example, patients with acute leukaemia may present with gingival bleeding as a result of thrombocytopenia (tumour infiltration of the bone marrow).[6]

Treatment-related problems

Anticancer treatments are associated with a variety of oral complications. Again, the oral problems may be the result of a direct effect of the treatment (e.g. mucositis), or an indirect effect of the treatment (e.g. infection).

Table 18.3 Oral complications of chemotherapy in paediatric patients[10]

Acute problems	Chronic problems
Mucositis	Maldevelopment of teeth
Salivary gland dysfunction	
Taste disturbance	
Oral infections, e.g. oral candidosis, HSV* infections, bacterial periapical infections	
Haemorrhage	

* HSV = herpes simplex virus

All children should have a thorough oral/dental assessment prior to the commencement of anticancer treatment. The aims of this assessment are:

1. To identify and treat sources of infection;

2. To identify and treat sources of irritation, e.g. broken restorations; and

3. To establish a suitable oral hygiene regimen.[7]

In some cases, patients will be prescribed additional agents to prevent/ameliorate specific complications of the treatment (e.g. mucositis, infections).

A number of guidelines have been produced on the oral care of patients undergoing anticancer treatment.[8,9] It should be noted that oral hygiene is discussed in detail in Chapter 3, whilst the management of specific complications of anticancer treatment is discussed in detail in Chapter 15.

Systemic chemotherapy

Systemic chemotherapy is frequently used in paediatric oncology. The oral complications of chemotherapy in children are shown in Table 18.3.[10] Chemotherapy-related oral problems are discussed further in Chapter 15.

Local radiotherapy

Local (head and neck) radiotherapy is less frequently used in paediatric oncology. However, total body irradiation will include head and neck irradiation (see below).[10] The complications of radiotherapy to the oral cavity in children are shown in Table 18.4. Radiotherapy-related oral problems are also discussed further in Chapter 15.

Bone marrow transplantation

Oral problems are common in patients that undergo a bone marrow transplant, and vary according to the stage of the bone marrow transplant (Table 18.5).[7] Many of these problems are related to the 'conditioning' regimen, which consists of systemic chemotherapy and/or total body irradiation.

Non-malignant disease

HIV infection/AIDS

The United Nations/WHO have estimated that there were 3.2 million children infected with HIV virus in 2002.[11] Moreover, they have estimated that 800,000 children

Table 18.4 Oral complications of radiotherapy in paediatric patients[10]

Acute problems	Chronic problems
Mucositis	Salivary gland dysfunction
Salivary gland dysfunction	Dental caries
Taste disturbance	Trismus
Oral infections, e.g. oral candidosis	Maldevelopment of teeth
	Maldevelopment of facial bones

contracted the infection, and that 610,000 children died from the infection, during 2002. The majority of cases are in Sub-Saharan Africa, but the infection is endemic in most parts of the world. In children, the most common mechanism of infection is vertical transmission, i.e. from mother to child (*in utero*, during birth, or during breastfeeding).

Oral problems are very common in HIV infection/AIDS.[12] Interestingly, the oral problems encountered in children are somewhat different from those encountered in adults. Table 16.2 shows the consensus classification of orofacial lesions associated with paediatric HIV infection.[13] It should be noted that the prevalence of most

Table 18.5 Oral complications of bone marrow transplantation. Adapted from reference [7]

Stage 1 Pre-transplant	Stage 2 Conditioning to early engraftment	Stage 3 Early engraftment to recovery of circulating counts	Stage 4 Recovery of circulating counts to immune reconstitution	Stage 5 Long term survival
See text	Mucositis	Mucositis	Infections	Xerostomia
	Infections	Infections	– fungal	Dental caries
	– fungal,	– fungal	– viral	Dental/skeletal
	e.g. oral	– viral	Xerostomia	growth and
	candidosis	– bacterial	Chronic	development
	– viral, e.g. HSV*	Xerostomia	GVHD**	problems
	– bacterial	Haemorrhage	Recurrence	Malignancy
	Xerostomia	GVHD**	malignancy	(secondary)
	Haemorrhage	– acute	Dental caries	
	Acute GVHD**	– chronic	Dental/skeletal	
		Recurrence	growth and	
		malignancy	development	
			problems	
			Malignancy	
			(secondary)	

*HSV = herpes simplex virus
**GVHD = graft versus host disease

oral problems has decreased since the introduction of highly active antiretroviral therapy (HAART). Nevertheless, oral problems are still seen at diagnosis, and at disease progression.

Oral problems in HIV infection/AIDS are discussed in detail in Chapter 16.

Organ transplantation

Oral problems are common in patients that have undergone a solid organ transplant, and are receiving maintenance immunosuppressive therapy. The oral problems encountered include infections (fungal, viral), malignancies (carcinomas, lymphomas) and miscellaneous other conditions (hairy leukoplakia, gingival hyperplasia).[14] Indeed, the oral problems encountered in this group of patients are not dissimilar to those encountered in patients with HIV infection.

Gingival hyperplasia is a relatively common side-effect of the immunosuppressive drug ciclosporin.[15] The pathophysiology of gingival hyperplasia is not well understood, although there does seem to be an association with the presence of dental plaque. It should be noted that gingival hyperplasia can also be a side-effect of phenytoin and nifedipine (and, to a lesser extent, other anticonvulsants/calcium antagonists).

Figure 18.4(a) demonstrates the clinical appearance of gingival hyperplasia. In addition to cosmetic issues, gingival hyperplasia may be associated with functional problems, e.g. difficulty chewing, difficulty speaking, problems with eruption of teeth.[15] Gingival hyperplasia may impair the ability to perform oral hygiene measures, which may lead to an increase in dental plaque (and an increase in gingival hyperplasia).

The management of gingival hyperplasia includes substitution of ciclosporin for another immunosuppressive drug (i.e. tacrolimus), good oral hygiene (tooth-brushing, chlorhexidine rinses, scaling, root planing), antibiotic therapy (i.e. azithromycin), and/or surgery (gingivectomy, periodontal flap).[15] It should be noted that surgery should only be undertaken once oral hygiene is at a satisfactory level.

The gingivectomy technique is a matter of personal choice. At the Great Ormond Street Hospital for Children the practice has been to use a surgical diathermy. The diathermy is used to excise the densely fibrous redundant gingivae, and then the tip of the diathermy is used to refine the contour of the gingivae.

The surgical area is covered with a periodontal dressing pack, which is removed about a week after the surgery. Initially, chlorhexidine rinses are used to control dental plaque. However, once healing is sufficiently advanced, toothbrushing should be reintroduced to the oral hygiene regimen (6–10 days). The results of treatment are highly satisfactory (Figs 18.4(a) and (b)).

Gingival hyperplasia tends to recur, unless the ciclosporin is discontinued.[15] Nevertheless, control of dental plaque will delay recurrence of gingival hyperplasia.

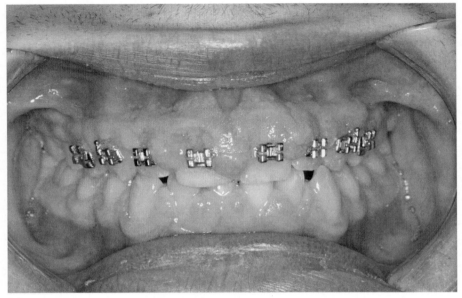

(a)

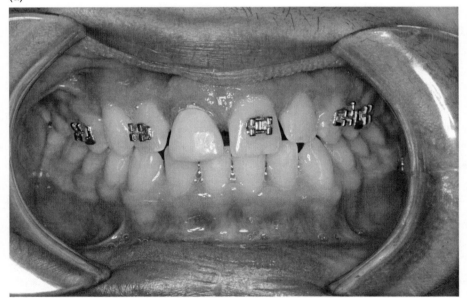

(b)

Fig. 18.4 (a) Gingival hyperplasia (pre-treatment). **(b)** Gingival hyperplasia (post-treatment).

Other non-malignant diseases

As discussed above, children with life-limiting conditions are at increased risk of developing typical paediatric dental problems, i.e. dental caries, periodontal disease.[16] However, children with life-limiting conditions may also develop a range of other oral/dental problems.[17,18] Some problems are relatively non-specific (e.g. drooling – patients with neuromuscular disorders),[19] whilst other problems are more specific (e.g. oral blistering – patients with epidermolysis bullosa).[20]

Cystic fibrosis[17,21]

Interestingly, children with cystic fibrosis are reported to have low levels of dental caries and periodontal disease. It is thought that this phenomenon relates to long-term antibiotic usage. However, children with cystic fibrosis are reported to have high levels of dental calculus, and enamel defects.

Duchenne muscular dystrophy[22,23]

The oral problems associated with this condition include macroglossia (enlargement of tongue), difficulty swallowing, and involuntary movements of orofacial muscles. Other reported abnormalities include delayed tooth eruption, and agenesis of the second premolar teeth.

Cerebral palsy[17,24]

Children with severe cerebral palsy are reported to have high levels of dental caries and periodontal disease. In addition, these children may develop malocclusion (protrusion of upper teeth), bruxism (grinding of teeth), difficulty chewing, difficulty swallowing, drooling, involuntary movements of the orofacial muscles, and temporomandibular joint dysfunction. Moreover, children with severe cerebral palsy are reported to have high levels of dental trauma.

References

1. Association for Children with Life-threatening or Terminal Conditions and their Families (ACT) and Royal College of Paediatrics and Child Health (2003). *A Guide to the Development of Children's Palliative Care Services*, 2nd edn. Bristol: ACT.

2. Harrison MG, Roberts GJ (1998). Comprehensive dental treatment of healthy and chronically sick children under intubation general anaesthesia during a 5-year period. *Br Dent J* **184**: 503–6.

3. Royal College of Paediatrics and Child Health and Neonatal and Paediatric Pharmacists Group (2003). *Medicines for Children*, 2nd edn. Poole: Direct Books.

4. Collins JJ, Byrnes ME, Dunkel IJ, Lapin J, Nadel T, Thaler HT *et al.* (2000). The measurement of symptoms in children with cancer. *J Pain Symptom Manage* **19**: 363–77.

5. Duggal MS, Curzon ME, Bailey CC, Lewis IJ, Prendergast M (1997). Dental parameters in the long term survivors of childhood cancer compared with siblings. *Oral Oncol* **33**: 348–53.

6. Laskaris G (2000). *Colour Atlas of Oral Diseases in Children and Adolescents*. Stuttgart: Georg Thieme Verlag.

7. Majorana A, Schubert MM, Porta F, Ugazio AG, Sapelli PL (2000). Oral complications of pediatric haematopoietic cell transplantation: diagnosis and management. *Support Care Cancer* **8**: 353–65.

8. Clinical Effectiveness Committee of the Faculty of Dental Surgery of the Royal College of Surgeons of England and British Society for Disability and Oral Health (2001). *Clinical Guidelines for the Oral Management of Oncology Patients Requiring Radiotherapy, Chemotherapy or Bone Marrow Transplantation Monograph on the Internet.* London: RCS and BDSH. Available from: http://www.rcseng.ac.uk/dental/fds/pdf/oncolradio.doc

9. National Cancer Institute (2004). *Oral Complications of Chemotherapy and Head/Neck Radiation Monograph on the Internet.* Bethesda: NCI. Available from: http://www.cancer.gov/cancerinfo/pdq/supportivecare/oralcomplications/HealthProfessional

10. Chin EA (1998). A brief overview of the oral complications in pediatric oncology patients and suggested management strategies. *J Dent Child* **65**: 468–73.

11. Joint United Nations Programme on HIV/AIDS (UNAIDS) and World Health Organization (WHO) (2002). *AIDS epidemic update: December 2002.* Geneva: UNAIDS and WHO.

12. Patton LL, Phelan JA, Ramos-Gomez FJ, Nittayananta W, Shiboski CH, Mbuguye TL (2002). Prevalence and classification of HIV-associated oral lesions. *Oral Dis* **8**, Suppl 2: 98–109.

13. Ramos-Gomez FJ, Flaitz C, Catapano P, Murray P, Milnes AR, Dorenbaum A (1999). Classification, diagnostic criteria, and treatment recommendations for orofacial manifestations in HIV-infected pediatric patients. Collaborative Workgroup on Oral Manifestations of Pediatric HIV Infection. *J Clin Pediatr Dent* **23**: 85–96.

14. Seymour RA, Thomason JM, Nolan A (1997). Oral lesions in organ transplant patients. *J Oral Pathol Med* **26**: 297–304.

15. Camargo PM, Melnick PR, Pirih FQ, Lagos R, Takei HH (2001). Treatment of drug-induced gingival enlargement: aesthetic and functional considerations. *Periodontol 2000* **27**: 131–8.

16. Tesini DA, Fenton SJ (1994). Oral health needs of persons with physical or mental disabilities. *Dent Clin North Am* **38**: 483–98.

17. McDonald RE, Avery DR (1994). *Dentistry for the Child and Adolescent,* 6th edn. St. Louis: Mosby.

18. Welbury RR (2001). *Paediatric Dentistry,* 2nd edn. Oxford: Oxford University Press.

19. Hussein I, Kershaw AE, Tahmassebi JF, Fayle SA (1998). The management of drooling in children and patients with mental and physical disabilities: a literature review. *Int J Paediatr Dent* **8**: 3–11.

20. Sedano HO, Gorlin RJ (1989). Epidermolysis bullosa. *Oral Surg Oral Med Oral Pathol* **67**: 555–63.

21. Narang A, Maguire A, Nunn JH, Bush A (2003). Oral health and related factors in cystic fibrosis and other chronic respiratory disorders. *Arch Dis Child* **88**: 702–7.

22. Morinushi T, Mastumoto S (1986). Oral findings and a proposal for a dental health care program for patients with Duchenne type muscular dystrophy. *Spec Care Dentist* **6**: 117–19.

23. Symons AL, Townsend GC, Hughes TE (2002). Dental characteristics of patients with Duchenne muscular dystrophy. *J Dent Child* **69**: 277–83.

24. Rodrigues dos Santos MT, Masiero D, Novo NF, Simionato MR (2003). Oral conditions in children with cerebral palsy. *J Dent Child (Chic)* **70**: 40–6.

Index